CURRENT CLINICAL PATHOLOGY

Antonio Giordano, MD, PhD
Philadelphia, PA, USA

Series Editor

More information about this series at http://www.springer.com/series/7632

Francesco M. Sacerdoti •
Antonio Giordano • Carlo Cavaliere
Editors

Advanced Imaging Techniques in Clinical Pathology

The original version of this book was revised. An erratum to the book can be found at DOI 10.1007/978-1-4939-3469-0_14.

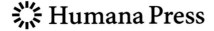 Humana Press

Editors
Francesco M. Sacerdoti
Temple University
College of Science and Technology
Philadelphia, PA
USA

Antonio Giordano
Temple University
College of Science and Technology
Philadelphia, PA
USA

Carlo Cavaliere
NAPLab – IRCCS SDN
Naples, Italy

ISSN 2197-781X   ISSN 2197-7828   (electronic)
Current Clinical Pathology
ISBN 978-1-4939-3467-6   ISBN 978-1-4939-3469-0   (eBook)
DOI 10.1007/978-1-4939-3469-0

Library of Congress Control Number: 2016950444

Printed on acid-free paper

This Humana Press imprint is published by Springer Nature
The registered company is Springer Science+Business Media LLC New York

Contents

List of Contributors

M. Aiello NAPLab – IRCCS SDN, Naples, Italy

Maria Paola Belfiore Sezione Scientifica di Radiodiagnostica, Radioterapia e Medicina Nucleare. Dipartimento Medico Chirurgico di Internistica Clinica e Sperimentale, "F. MAGRASSI" e "A. LANZARA", Seconda Università degli Studi di Napoli, Naples, Italy

D. Berritto Sezione Scientifica di Radiodiagnostica, Radioterapia e Medicina Nucleare. Dipartimento Medico Chirurgico di Internistica Clinica e Sperimentale "F. MAGRASSI" e "A. LANZARA", Seconda Università degli Studi di Napoli, Naples, Italy

Angelina Di Carlo Department of Medico Surgical Sciences and Biotechnologies, University of Rome "Sapienza," Corso della Repubblica, Latina, Italy

C. Cavaliere NAPLab – IRCCS SDN, Naples, Italy

Letizia Cito INT-CROM, "Pascale Foundation" National Cancer Institute-Cancer Research Center, Mercogliano, Italy

Vincenzo Cuccurullo Sezione Scientifica di Radiodiagnostica, Radioterapia e Medicina Nucleare. Dipartimento Medico Chirurgico di Internistica Clinica e Sperimentale "F. MAGRASSI" e "A. LANZARA", Seconda Università degli Studi di Napoli, Naples, Italy

Vincenzo Desiderio Dipartimento di Medicina Sperimentale, Sezione di Biotecnologie, Istologia Medica e Biologia Molecolare, Seconda Università degli Studi di Napoli, Napoli, Italy

Marina Di Domenico Department of Biochemistry, Biophysics and General Pathology, Seconda Università degli Studi di Napoli, Naples, Italy

Antonia Feola Department of Biology, University of Naples, Naples, Italy

A. Giordano Temple University, Philadelphia, PA, USA

Alfonso Giovane Department of Biochemistry, Biophysics and General Pathology, Seconda Università degli Studi di Napoli, Naples, Italy

Roberto Grassi Sezione Scientifica di Radiodiagnostica, Radioterapia e Medicina Nucleare. Dipartimento Medico Chirurgico di Internistica Clinica e Sperimentale "F. MAGRASSI" e "A. LANZARA", Seconda Università degli Studi di Napoli, Naples, Italy

Graziella Di Grezia Sezione Scientifica di Radiodiagnostica, Radioterapia e Medicina Nucleare. Dipartimento Medico Chirurgico di Internistica Clinica e Sperimentale, "F. MAGRASSI" e "A. LANZARA", Seconda Università degli Studi di Napoli, Naples, Italy

F. Iacobellis Sezione Scientifica di Radiodiagnostica, Radioterapia e Medicina Nucleare. Dipartimento Medico Chirurgico di Internistica Clinica e Sperimentale "F. MAGRASSI" e "A. LANZARA", Seconda Università degli Studi di Napoli, Naples, Italy

D. De Luca U.O. Fisica Sanitaria, Lecce, Italy

Luigi Mansi Sezione Scientifica di Radiodiagnostica, Radioterapia e Medicina Nucleare. Dipartimento Medico Chirurgico di Internistica Clinica e Sperimentale "F. MAGRASSI" e "A. LANZARA", Seconda Università degli Studi di Napoli, Naples, Italy

L. Marcello Institute of Human Anatomy, Seconda Università degli Studi di Napoli, Naples, Italy

V. Mollo Center for Advanced Biomaterials for Health Care CABHC, Istituto Italiano di Tecnologia, Naples, Italy

P.A. Netti Center for Advanced Biomaterials for Health Care CABHC - Istituto Italiano di Tecnologia, Naples, Italy

CRIB – Centro di Ricerca Interdipartimentale sui Biomateriali – Università Federico II di Napoli, Naples, Italy

Francesca Paino Dipartimento di Medicina Sperimentale, Sezione di Biotecnologie, Istologia Medica e Biologia Molecolare, Seconda Università degli Studi di Napoli, Napoli, Italy

Gianpaolo Papaccio Dipartimento di Medicina Sperimentale, Sezione di Biotecnologie, Istologia Medica e Biologia Molecolare, Seconda Università degli Studi di Napoli, Napoli, Italy

V. Parlato Department of Radiological Sciences, Seconda Università degli Studi di Napoli, Naples, Italy

Michele La Rocca University of Salerno, Fisciano SA, Italy

Claudia Rossi Sezione Scientifica di Radiodiagnostica, Radioterapia e Medicina Nucleare. Dipartimento Medico Chirurgico di Internistica Clinica e Sperimentale, "F. MAGRASSI" e "A. LANZARA", Seconda Università degli Studi di Napoli, Naples, Italy

Antonio Rotondo Sezione Scientifica di Radiodiagnostica, Radioterapia e Medicina Nucleare. Dipartimento Medico Chirurgico di Internistica Clinica e Sperimentale, "F. MAGRASSI" e "A. LANZARA", Seconda Università degli Studi di Napoli, Naples, Italy

Francesco M. Sacerdoti Temple University, Philadelphia, PA, USA

N. Pignatelli di Spinazzola Department of Radiological Sciences, Seconda Università degli Studi di Napoli, Naples, Italy

Virginia Tirino Dipartimento di Medicina Sperimentale, Sezione di Biotecnologie, Istologia Medica e Biologia Molecolare, Seconda Università degli Studi di Napoli, Napoli, Italy

E. Torino Center for Advanced Biomaterials for Health Care CABHC, Istituto Italiano di Tecnologia, Naples, Italy

Introduction

F.M. Sacerdoti and A. Giordano

This book was born of close collaboration between Professor Antonio Giordano— a highly regarded pathologist—and Professor F.M. Sacerdoti, an engineer specializing in the realization of complex equipment and vision systems.

We agreed that pathologists, biologists, medical doctors, applied researchers, and others who work with imaging systems, such as microscopes, time-to-amplitude converter, etc., every day, would benefit from a deeper understanding of how these systems work, what software can be used to process their information, why the image is so confusing, and so on.

The first chapter is a basic guide to statistics, which is important for all working in the health field. We then provide an overview of the latest techniques in several medical fields, from pathology, microscopy, and cytometry to advanced microscopy techniques.

Each chapter has been prepared by an expert in the field—someone who works with the specific topic on a daily basis—to provide realistic insight into the techniques, their use, and specific lessons learned.

F.M. Sacerdoti (✉) • A. Giordano
Temple University, Philadelphia, PA, USA
e-mail: sacerdoti@e-voluzione.it; giordano@temple.edu

© Springer Science+Business Media New York 2016
F.M. Sacerdoti et al. (eds.), *Advanced Imaging Techniques in Clinical Pathology*,
Current Clinical Pathology, DOI 10.1007/978-1-4939-3469-0_1

Part I

Basic Knowledge

Digital Image Processing

2

Francesco M. Sacerdoti

Scope

The scope of this introductory chapter is to provide the reader with the basic definitions and information necessary to easily understand the rest of the book and to use digital image processing systems and software.

Techniques

Introduction

Digital image processing is the acquisition of an image from the real world, followed by its processing and analysis (see Fig. 2.1). For more detailed information see [1] and [2].

Image Acquisition

An image from the real world is captured via an image acquisition system, which transforms the light information (or X-ray or other signals) into a digital image.

Image Processing

The digital image is then improved by enhancing the contrast, details, colors, and other characteristics.

Image Analysis

Starting with the digital image, image analysis extracts all parts and characteristics of the image. This module also creates all the necessary results: features, pictures, and measures.

The term "features" refers to all the characteristics of the image specific to the analysis being conducted.

"Feature extraction" is a primary element of image analysis software. For example, it extracts all small images of cells present in the entire image to allow for subsequent counting or measuring.

"Pictures" are all the graphical outputs, for example, an X-ray picture, useful for subsequent human analysis done by the physician.

"Measure" is a list of necessary measurements to be taken from the image, such as fetal length in echo-imaging.

An example is shown in Fig. 2.2.

1. The image from the real world is acquired using some hardware, in this example, a simple photo camera.
2. The image is acquired with acquisition software that transforms the real image into pixels (see inside the *circle*).
3. The image processing software processes the image, enhancing the image quality by, for example, enhancing contrast.
4. The image analysis software extracts important information from the image. The figure shows the extraction of water from the image.

F.M. Sacerdoti (✉)
Temple University, Philadelphia, PA, USA
e-mail: sacerdoti@e-voluzione.it

© Springer Science+Business Media New York 2016
F.M. Sacerdoti et al. (eds.), *Advanced Imaging Techniques in Clinical Pathology*,
Current Clinical Pathology, DOI 10.1007/978-1-4939-3469-0_2

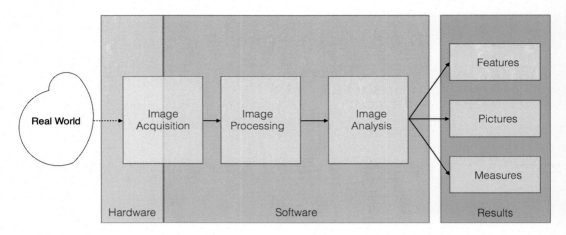

Fig. 2.1 Image analysis principles

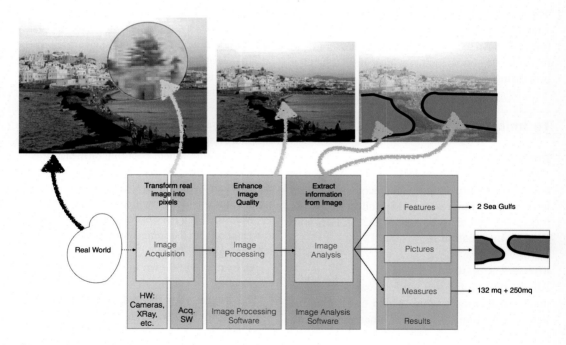

Fig. 2.2 Example of image analysis

5. The results from the image analysis software are the features, pictures, and measures (described as follows).

Basic Concepts

To simplify our descriptions, from now on we refer solely to images from light sources (e.g., microscope or digital camera), but the concept is also the same if the images come from other sources such as X-rays, acoustic images, etc.

Digital Image

The output of a camera is a matrix $N \times M$ of pixels normally called "digital image."

Pixel

The "pixel" is the smallest item in a digital image. Each pixel is a sample of an original image obtained by the image acquisition system; more pixels means more accurate representation of the original image.

If you zoom in on a digital image, the pixel may be seen as a dot. It has two features: coordinates (x,y) and value (v). The coordinates univocally identify a single pixel and they are the indexes of the pixel inside the matrix.

The data type of v changes depending on the type of digital image:

> *Grayscale Image*
> The value of each pixel in a grayscale image is usually represented by a number—from 0 to 255—that represents the intensity of the light at that point. A value of 255 means white, whereas a value of 0 is black. Some systems use a more precise grayscale representation, with more values to represent the light intensity (e.g., 0–4095 [12-bit image] or 0–65535 [16-bit image]).
>
> *Color Image*
> In color images, a pixel is typically a triple of gray components (red, green, and blue intensities) or, less frequently, four components (cyan, magenta, yellow, and black intensities). The latter is used more often in printing than in image analysis. Each "plane" (red, green, and blue) is usually treated as a single gray image for feature extraction.

Pixel Resolution

Resolution is the capability of the sensor to observe or measure the smallest object clearly with distinct boundaries. Resolution depends upon the size of the pixel.

With any given lens setting, the smaller the pixel, the higher the resolution and the clearer the object in the image will be. Images with smaller pixel sizes might consist of more pixels. The number of pixels correlates to the amount of information within the image.

The figure illustrates how the same image might appear at different pixel resolutions if the pixels were poorly rendered as sharp squares (a smooth image reconstruction from pixels is preferred, but the sharp squares better illustrate our point).

(source: public domain) (Fig. 2.3)

Acquisition

Several methods are available with which to transfer a digital image to a computer for further processing; the method usually depends on the specific hardware used. The most common systems are via Ethernet (which does not require the installation of specific drivers; instead, the IP address of the camera must be set to match that of the computer) or a USB connection (which do require the installation of a specific driver).

Another interface that is becoming more common, especially in recent years, is FireWire, which requires a specific computer card.

More information follows on specific image hardware.

Image Processing

Image processing is used to enhance the quality of the original image; the process used depends mainly on what the image analysis must find or measure within the image. Specific algorithms are applied to the whole image or a part of it. Examples are as follows:

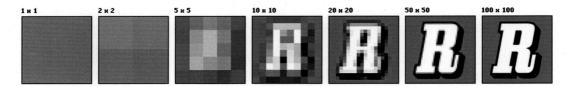

Fig. 2.3 Example of pixel resolution

- *Crop*: Cropping creates a new image by selecting a desired rectangular portion from the image being cropped. The unwanted part of the image is discarded. Image cropping does not reduce the resolution of the area cropped.
- *Noise reduction:* The purpose is to remove, without loss of detail, "noise" due to conditions such as poor light or extreme zooming. Excessive noise reduction leads to a loss of detail; its application is hence subject to a trade-off between the undesirability of the noise itself and that of the reduction artifacts.
- *Lens correction*: Within the characteristics of the optic system used, lens correction allows the user to compensate for various lens distortions.
- *Enhancing images*: Enhancing is used to make an image lighter or darker or to increase or decrease contrast. Some examples are shown in Figs. 2.4 and 2.5

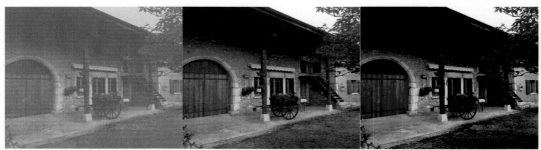

Low Contrast   Good Contrast   High Contrast

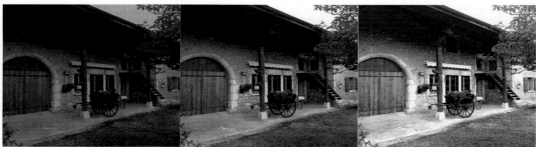

Low Exposure   Good Exposure   High Exposure

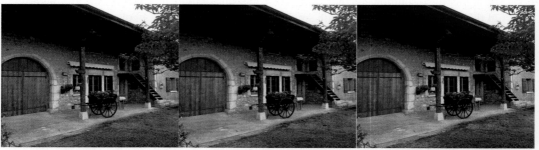

Low Saturation   Good Saturation   High Saturation

Fig. 2.4 Example of image processing

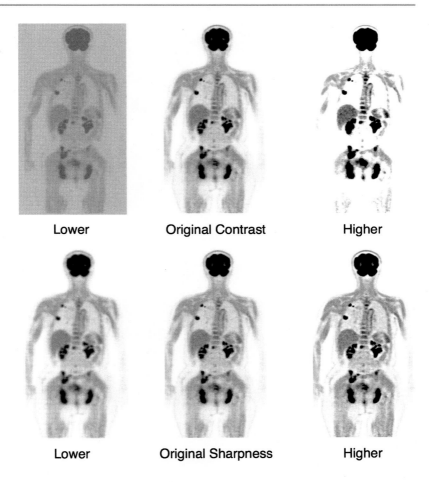

Fig. 2.5 Comparison between contrast and sharpness

- *Sharpening and softening:* This kind of processing enables the user to sharpen and blur images in a number of ways, such as unsharp masking and deconvolution. Another similar and useful technique is "edge enhancement," with which the contrast can be increased at sharp changes in color inside the image.
- *Histogram analysis*: This analysis starts with creating the distribution of pixel values by counting the number of similar pixels. Some examples are shown in Fig. 2.6.
  Histogram analysis enables operations such as the following examples:
  - *Inverse:* Exchange bright pixels with dark pixels.
  - *Equalize:* Create an image with an equal number of bright and dark pixels.
  - *Threshold:* Every pixel with a value higher (or lower) than a set threshold is transformed into black (or white). This technique is useful when extracting specific characteristics or areas from the image.
- *Filtering*: Complete libraries of filters are available for application to an image to enhance, for example, shadow pixels, or to sharpen edges. See the references for more information.
- *Color image processing:* Some techniques are dedicated to color images. For example, it is possible to extract a single plane from a color

Fig. 2.6 Histograms

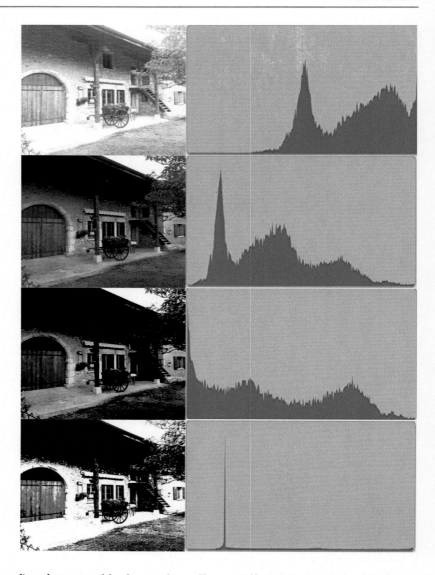

image (e.g., blue or red) and process this single image as grayscale.

Image Analysis

The next step is the analysis of the image.

In several fields, applications may be completely automatic. However, this is not possible in medical fields, as human analysis is always necessary. Image analysis can help measure objects and recognize features, among others. Every different application performs a different analysis.

Some examples of analysis are as follows:

- *Image segmentation*: The process of partitioning a digital image into multiple segments is known as image segmentation. The goal of this function is to simplify the representation of an image into something more meaningful and easier to analyze. Image segmentation is typically used to locate objects and boundaries (lines, curves, etc.) in images. Image segmentation assigns a label to every pixel, taking into account its characteristics and those of the neighboring pixels (color, luminance, differences, distance from image border, etc.). Thus, all pixels with the same characteristics are allocated the same label.

- *False color analysis*: This technique transforms the pixel using specific color scales to highlight image characteristics. A simple example is thermography, which normally uses a scale called "fire" (based on yellows and reds) to highlight a specific range of temperatures in the body under analysis. Thermographic analyses are used in medicine to diagnose a range of diseases such as breast cancer, thyroid function, muscle and joint inflammation, microcirculation problems, or fibromyalgia. The false color image shows the distribution of temperatures on the part of the body analyzed, highlighting differences in temperature that may be caused by disease.

- *2D and 3D object recognition*: This technique finds and identifies objects in images or video sequences. Whereas humans easily recognize a multitude of objects in images with little effort (also with different viewpoints, sizes, and scales; translated or rotated), it remains a challenge for computer vision systems.

- *Pattern recognition:* In medical fields, it is important to recognize "patterns" inside an image, for example, identifying different tissues in an echography. Pattern recognition is a branch of machine learning that focuses on the recognition of patterns and regularities in data. The systems are typically trained with labeled "training" data, and the system then searches for similar patterns in the image.

- *Motion detection:* This process detects a change in the position of an object relative to its surroundings or a change in the surroundings relative to an object. For example, in medicine, motion detection could track particles to follow how one cell moves with respect to others in a cell culture.

Software

We provide in the following, a preliminary list of software useful for image acquisition, processing, and analysis, with links for further information. Obviously, this list cannot be complete and we apologize if we have missed any. All software names and brand names are the property of their respective owners, and the example images have been reproduced from the corresponding websites or brochures.

General Purpose
LabVIEW with IMAQ add-on: http://www.ni.com

LabVIEW is a complete programming language environment for the acquisition, processing, and analysis of signals, images, image sequences, and videos. In particular, it includes one of the most complete sets in the world for image acquisition, processing, and analysis (IMAQ). There is also a plug-in dedicated to BioSignal processing and medical applications that allows, for example, the use of DICOM (Digital Imaging and Communications in Medicine) and DICOMDIR/IMGDIR images.

MATLAB with Image Processing Toolbox: http://ch.mathworks.com/products/image/

Image Processing Toolbox™ provides a comprehensive set of reference-standard algorithms, functions, and applications for image processing, analysis, visualization, and algorithm development. MATLAB can perform image analysis, image segmentation, image enhancement, noise reduction, geometric transformations, and image registration.

Halcon: http://www.halcon.com

Halcon is a general-purpose image processing and machine vision software with a large library of more than 2000 operators for low-, medium-, and high-level image processing.

ImageJ: http://imagej.nih.gov/ij

ImageJ is a complete software continuously enriched with plug-ins to process and analyze images. It is written in Java and is therefore multiplatform. Most software are compatible with ImageJ.

Icy: http://icy.bioimageanalysis.org

Icy is an open community platform for bioimaging informatics created by the Quantitative Image Analysis Unit at Institut Pasteur. It includes the primary software and more than 300 plug-ins.

Image-Pro Plus: http://www.mediacy.com/ index.aspx?page=IPP

Image-Pro Plus image analysis software enables the user to acquire images; count, measure, and classify objects; and automate work. It offers automated microscope control, image capture, measurement, count/size, and macro development tools.

Microscopy Image acquisition

Micromanager: https://www.micro-manager. org/

µManager is a software package for the control of automated microscopes. It is compatible with ImageJ.

ScanImage: http://vidriotechnologies.com
by Vijay Iyer, Karel Swoboda

This software enables the control of experiments using two-photon laser scanning microscopy. Vidrio develops software to facilitate complex cellular in vivo imaging experiments. It is used mainly in neuroscience imaging.

Display and Segmentation

Vaa3D: http://home.penglab.com/proj/vaa3d/ home/index.html

Vaa3D visualizes and explores large 3D/4D/ 5D images, extracts complex surface objects from images, and performs comprehensive analyses such as brain connectome mapping. It can render 5D (spatial-temporal) data directly in the 3D volume-rendering mode.

BioimageXD: http://www.bioimagexd.net

BioImageXD is a free open-source software package for the analysis, processing, and visualization of multidimensional microscopy images. It is a collaborative project between the universities of Jyväskylä and Turku in Finland, the Max Planck Institute CBG in Dresden, Germany, and collaborators worldwide. BioImageXD is a multipurpose post-processing tool for bioimaging that can be used for simple

visualization of multichannel temporal image stacks to complex 3D rendering of multiple channels at once.

VisBio: http://loci.wisc.edu/software/visbio

VisBio is a biological visualization tool designed for easy visualization and analysis of multidimensional image data developed by Curtis Rueden and Abraham Sorber at the University of Wisconsin–Madison Laboratory for Optical and Computational Instrumentation (LOCI).

Image Processing
COSMOS: http://cirl.memphis.edu/cosmos. php

The Computational Optical Sectioning Microscopy Open Source (COSMOS) software package is currently under development by the Computational Imaging Research Laboratory (CIRL) led by Dr. Preza. COSMOS has four platform-independent graphical user interfaces (GUIs) developed using a visualization tool kit for Point Spread Function (PSF) generation, intensity estimation, image visualization, and performance analysis.

3D_Deconvolution: http://bigwww.epfl.ch/ algorithms/deconvolutionlab/

By Cédric Vonesch, Raquel Terrés Cristofani, and Guillaume Schmit at the Biomedical Image Group (BIG), EPFL, Switzerland

DeconvolutionLab is a software package (ImageJ plug-in) to deconvolve 2D or 3D microscopic images based on the knowledge of the PSF. It implements a variety of deconvolution algorithms and includes a convolution tool to generate simulated datasets with additive noise.

OptiNav: http://www.optinav.com/imagej. html

This site makes available ImageJ plug-ins and macros and MATLAB scripts for several image processing techniques that are also applicable to biomedical imaging.

Voxx: http://www.indiana.edu/~voxx/

Voxx is a voxel-based (not surface-based) 3D-rendering program that has been optimized for biological microscopy. This software permits researchers to perform real-time rendering of large microscopy datasets using inexpensive personal computers. It was developed primarily to explore 3D datasets collected on confocal and multiphoton microscopy systems.

CellProfiler and CellProfiler Analyst: http://www.cellprofiler.org

by Ann Carpenter, MIT

CellProfiler cell image analysis software is designed for biologists without training in computer vision or programming to quantitatively measure phenotypes from thousands of images automatically.

CellProfiler Analyst allows interactive exploration and analysis of data, particularly from high-throughput, image-based experiments. Included is a supervised machine-learning system that can be trained to recognize complicated and subtle phenotypes for automatic scoring of millions of cells.

IVE and Priism: http://www.msg.ucsf.edu/IVE/index.html

Priism is a collection of tools for processing, analyzing, and visualizing multidimensional imagery with a focus on 3D wide-field optical microscopy and electron microscopy Electron Microscopy (EM) tomography. The image visualization environment (IVE) forms the core set of software libraries that are the foundation for the tools in Priism.

Cell Tracking

CellTracker: http://dbkgroup.org/celltracker/

CellTracker is a free software environment for image browsing, processing, and cell tracking that enables the user to track targets in living cell imaging.

View5D: http://www.nanoimaging.de/View5D/

Java Applet, ImageJ plug-in, MATLAB plug-in.

The program View5D interactively displays up to five dimension volumetric datasets.

Multidimensional data frequently arise in confocal microscopy and medical imaging applications. The program includes three orthogonal slicing views, 2D and 3D histograms of intensity (scattergrams), basic image processing operations, interactive counting and tagging of entities, tracking of 3D movements, and multiplicative display of lifetime or ratio images.

OME (Open Microscopy Environment): www.openmicroscopy.org/

OME provides data management for biological light microscopy, image-based analysis of cellular dynamics, and image-based screens of cellular localization or phenotypes. It is a database engine that enables a laboratory to store all microscopy images along with metadata, thus keeping track of projects.

DIPimage/DIPlib: http://www.diplib.org

DIPimage is a MATLAB toolbox for scientific image processing and analysis. It is a tool for teaching and research in image processing.

DIPlib is a platform-independent scientific image processing library written in C. It has a large number of functions for processing and analyzing multidimensional image data. The library provides functions for performing transformations, filter operations, object generation, local structure analysis, object measurements, and statistical analysis of images. Key design features include ample support for different data types (binary, integer, floating point, complex) and dimensionalities.

References[1]

1. Gonzalez RC, Woods RE. Digital image processing. 2nd ed. Upper Saddle River, NJ: Prentice Hall; 2001.
2. Russ JC. The image processing handbook, ISBN 0-8493-7254-2 (2006).

[1] These references are general texts for studying image processing and analysis.

Statistical Analysis and Software

3

Michele La Rocca

Scope

Statistics is the science of collecting, summarizing, analyzing, presenting, and interpreting data for decision making under uncertainty. Statistics allows "learning from experience" and plays a central role in biomedical research. Statistical tools are necessary to (1) decide how data should be collected; (2) decide how the collected data should be analyzed and summarized; and (3) measure the accuracy of the data summary. This latter step is part of the inference process, where the results of the statistical analysis allow the researcher to make some general statement about a wider set of subjects. All these three basic statistical concepts (data collection, summary, and inference) are deeply embedded in any research workflow.

Textbooks for the application of statistics in biomedical research are plentiful. The works by Altman [1] and Kirkwood and Sterne [2] are very good primers. A more technical yet still very accessible textbook is the work by Wayne [3]. For general and useful references, including discussion of several modern statistical techniques, see also the works by Wilcox [4–6].

Techniques

Some Basic Concepts

Statistical tools are useful for studying, analyzing, and learning about populations. A "population" is a set of statistical units. In statistics, the word "population" is used in a much wider sense than usual. It is not simply limited to a group of people but can refer to any collection of objects that is of interest for statistical research.

In studying a population, the focus can be on one or more "variables," in other words, on characteristics of the units of the population. Examples include the sex of a patient, blood pressure, or age. Variables are "measured" on the units of a well defined population and the measurement results are usually referred to as (raw) data. Measurement is the process by which numbers or attributes are assigned to a variable of single population units.

The first step in choosing the best statistical tool to use for learning from the data is to classify the variables into their different types, as different statistical methods pertain to each and can be considered as appropriate.

Variables are usually classified with respect to the type of measurement process as "quantitative" or "categorical." Quantitative variables are the result of numerical measurements and can be continuous or discrete. A continuous variable is

M. La Rocca (✉)
University of Salerno, Salerno, Italy
e-mail: larocca@unisa.it

© Springer Science+Business Media New York 2016
F.M. Sacerdoti et al. (eds.), *Advanced Imaging Techniques in Clinical Pathology*,
Current Clinical Pathology, DOI 10.1007/978-1-4939-3469-0_3

measured on a continuous scale (such as blood pressure), whereas a discrete variable can only take discrete values, usually whole numbers (such as the number of patients with a specific disease). Categorical variables are non-numerical data that can take on one of a fixed number of possible values. They can be further classified as nominal or ordinal. A nominal variable is the result of measurements that classify the statistical units into categories (such as ethnic group), whereas ordinal variables are the result of measurements that enable the units to be ordered with respect to the variable of interest (such as social class, which has a natural order, from poorest to richest). Important subsets of categorical variables are binary (or dichotomous) variables, which can take on only two alternative values (e.g., the sex of a subject [male or female] or the status of a patient [surviving or dead]). In many cases, the variables of interest are not directly measured but derived from those originally recorded via simple transformations (e.g., age can be derived from the date of birth).

Variables can also be classified with respect to the role they play in the statistical analysis. The "outcome" variable is the focus of the analysis, the variation or occurrence of which is to be understood. Often, the main interest is in identifying factors or "exposure" variables that may influence and explain the variability of the outcome variable. Depending on the context, outcome variables are also referred to as "response" or "dependent" variables, whereas exposure variables are also referred to as explanatory or independent variables. Again, depending on the context, different terms for the same type of variables are possible. For example, in clinical trials, the exposure is the treatment group; in case–control studies, the outcome is the case–control status and the exposure variables are known as risk factors.

An "observational" or an "experimental" research design can be used to collect data. In an observational design, data are collected about one or more groups of subjects, but nothing is done to affect these subjects. Observational designs can be "prospective" (observations are collected about events after the start of the study) or "retrospective" (observations are collected about past events and can be gathered from existing sources). Observational designs include censuses, surveys, case–control studies, and cohort studies. In a retrospective case–control design, a group of subjects (cases) with the condition of interest (e.g., a disease) is identified along with a group of unaffected subjects (controls), and their past exposure to one or more factors is then compared. If the cases report greater exposure than the controls, one can infer that exposure is causally related to the condition of interest. In a prospective "cohort" design, a group of subjects is identified and followed into the future. The cohort may also be subdivided at the beginning into groups with different characteristics to investigate which subjects enter a particular state (e.g., a disease). On the other hand, "experimental" designs are those where the researcher influences the events and investigates the effects of the intervention. A design can also be classified as "longitudinal" (used to investigate changes over time, possibly in relation to an intervention) or "cross-sectional" (subjects are observed only once). The book by Machin and Campbell [7] and the references therein are excellent references for design studies in biomedical science.

If a population is small, it is feasible to study all its units. However, populations of interest in biomedical applications are typically quite large, involving many (possibly thousands of) units. Moreover, in some cases, the measurement process is destructive for the statistical units (think of measuring the lifetime of a piece of equipment). In all these cases, just a "sample" (i.e., a subset) of the population units is studied. The method of selecting the sample is called the "sampling procedure." One very important sampling plan is "random sampling," which ensures that every subset of units in the population has the same chance of being included in the sample. This scheme ensures that the sample so selected is able to reproduce all the main characteristics of the population under study. However, more complex sampling designs can be used to improve the efficiency and the accuracy of the inference process (see Tillé [8] and the references therein).

Once a sample has been selected and the variables of interest measured for every sampled unit, the information contained in the sample is used to make an "inference" about the population. A statistical inference is an estimate, a prediction, or any other generalization about a population based on the information contained in a sample (a small subset of the population) to learn about the larger population. Clearly, the inference process is effective only if the sample correctly reproduces the main characteristics of the population under study. Note that, because of chance, selecting different samples from the population gives different sampling values; this must be taken into account when using a sample to make inferences about the population. This phenomenon, known as "sampling variability," lies at the very heart of any inference procedure.

Descriptive and Exploratory Tools

An essential (and often underestimated) step in statistical analysis is exploratory data analysis, where appropriate usage of summary measures and graphical tools can provide invaluable insight into the structure of the data and in identifying outliers (unusual values of a variable), possible errors in the data, and useful data transformation to meet required assumptions. This step gives the researcher insights into the location of the distribution (the tendency of the data to center about certain numerical values), the spread of the data (variability about the location), and the shape of the distribution. Those insights can be achieved via clever use of both numerical and graphical tools and are fundamental for a reliable application of more complex inferential and modeling tools.

Summarizing the Distribution of a Dataset
Let $y_1, y_2, \cdots, y_n$ be observations on a variable Y gathered using a sample of size n from the given population under study. The location of the distribution of the variable Y is the central tendency of the data, that is, the tendency of the data to center about certain numerical values. This important aspect of distributions can be measured using different tools chosen with respect to the type of data at hand.

If Y is a quantitative variable, the most common and best-understood measure of central tendency is the "arithmetic mean," which is simply the sum of all the observations in the sample divided by the sample size. It is defined as

$$\overline{y} = \frac{1}{n}\sum_{i=1}^{n} y_i$$

The mean has several nice properties, but it can be very misleading if outlying observations affect the data. Even a single extreme observation can completely destroy the ability of the mean to deliver the "centre" of the dataset. When the researcher suspects the dataset contains outliers, it is better to use a robust (resistant) statistical index, that is, summary measures designed to produce accurate results even if outliers are present.

A robust location index is the "median," defined as the midway value when the data are ranked in ascending order: by definition, half the distribution lies below the median and half above. Clearly, when the distribution of the data is approximately symmetric and there are no outliers, the mean and median are very close to each other. Similarly, the "lower quartile" (denoted by Q_1) is defined as the value below which 25 % of the values of the distribution lie, while the "upper quartile" (Q_3) is defined as the value below which 75 % of the values of the distribution lie. The quartiles, together with the median, divide the distribution into four equally sized groups.

When dealing with statistical indexes, an important property to characterize their robustness properties is the "breakdown point." It is defined as the fraction of extreme (large or small) observations that a statistical index can handle before giving arbitrary results. Thus, the larger the breakdown point of an index, the more robust it is. The breakdown point of the mean is equal to zero (a single outlying value can destroy the index), whereas that of the median is equal to

50 % (at most, 50 % of the data can be outliers without affecting its value). It is easy to see that the breakdown point of the quartiles is 25 %.

Nevertheless, medians have their drawbacks. Since not all information present in the sample is used to compute the median, this index is clearly less efficient than the mean. Robust location indexes more efficient than the median are the "midhinge" (the arithmetic mean of the two quartiles), the "truncated mean" (the mean of the observations after a fraction of the highest and lower values have been discarded), the "winsorized mean" (the mean of the data where extreme values are replaced by values closer to the median) (see Rosenberger and Gasko [9]).

Measures of central tendency provide only a partial description of a quantitative dataset, and the information would not be complete without a measure of the "variability" of the observations.

The simplest measure of variability is the "range" of the dataset, defined as the difference between the largest and smallest observations. This measure is quite crude and clearly not robust, but it is very simple to calculate and gives a very first idea of the range of variation of the observations, making it a useful tool for data checking.

The most popular measure for variability is the "standard deviation" (SD), defined as the square root of the "sample variance," that is, $s = \sqrt{s^2}$ where

$$s^2 = \frac{1}{n-1} \sum_{i=1}^{n} (y_i - \bar{y})^2$$

Clearly, both the variance and the standard deviation are not robust indexes with a zero breakdown point: a single outlier can destroy them.

Alternative robust measures are the "interquartile range," defined as the distance between the lower and the upper quartile $IQR = Q_3 - Q_1$ and the median absolute deviation (MAD), defined as

$$\text{MAD} = \text{Median}\{|y_i - \text{Median}\{y_i\}|\}$$

where |.| denotes absolute values. There is an approximate relationship between the MAD and the standard deviation, namely, $s = 1.4826\,\text{MAD}$. It can be shown that the breakdown point of the interquartile range is equal to 25 %, whereas that of the MAD is equal to 50 %. However, although the MAD is easy to compute, it suffers from a low efficiency. Alternative robust measures for spread that are more efficient than the MAD are given in Croux and Rousseeuw [10] and in Rousseeuw and Croux [11].

An effective and concise summary of the distribution of a single sample is the "five-number summary," obtained by reporting the sample minimum, the lower quartile, the median, the upper quartile, and the sample maximum. This summary gives information about the location (from the median), spread (from the interquartile range), and range (from the minimum and the maximum) of the observations. It also allows for a quick comparison of several sets of observations and has a very straightforward graphical representation, the box-and-whisker plot.

Data Checking and Outlier Identification

Outliers are observations that appear to be inconsistent with the majority of the data. This type of observation is often a problem in statistical analysis. By definition, they are extreme, and their inclusion or exclusion can lead to model misspecification, biased parameter estimation, and, in general, incorrect results (see Horn et al. [12], among others). However, please note that not all extreme values are outliers. An outlier has a low probability of originating from the same statistical distribution as the other observations in the dataset. On the other hand, an extreme value is an observation that might have a low probability of occurrence but cannot be statistically shown to originate from a different distribution than the rest of the data.

Outliers can arise from several different causes. Outliers can be (1) due to gross errors (such as human errors, instrumental and measurement errors, incorrect data entry, missing value codes used as real data); (2) generated as the result of the natural variation of population that cannot be controlled (these values are drawn from the intended population, but their values are unusual compared with the normal values); (3) due to sampling errors (i.e., not members of the population under study).

Not all outliers are illegitimate contaminants, and not all illegitimate values show up as outliers. Consequently, it is not always reasonable to remove outliers form the analysis simply because they appear to be extreme values. If they are not the result of some registration error, they could even be the focus of the statistical analysis (e.g., when looking for subjects with unusual behavior). In any case, it is always important to identify them prior to any statistical analysis and any modeling procedure.

The detection of outliers in univariate datasets can be pretty easy and can be based on the quartiles. The so-called Tukey fences give the thresholds for outlier detection. For lower outliers, the threshold is given by $Q_1 - 1.5(Q_3 - Q_1)$, whereas the threshold for upper outliers is given by $Q_3 + 1.5(Q_3 - Q_1)$. Observed values outside this interval are considered outliers. However, whereas it can be easy to spot extreme values in univariate data, it can be very difficult to spot them in multivariate datasets because of masking effects. Several statistical techniques have been developed to detect outliers in multivariate datasets. Technical details can be found in Barnett and Lewis [13] and in Atkinson et al. [14] and the references therein, whereas a shorter review can be found in Hadi et al. [15]. See also Solberg and Lahti [16] and Hodge and Austin [17] for a literature review from a machine-learning viewpoint and Fritsch et al. [18] for a very interesting review on outlier detection in medical imaging datasets.

Once outliers have been identified, the problem becomes how to deal with them. Basically, what to do depends on why an outlier is in the data. When outliers are the result of gross errors or registration errors, there is general agreement that those data points should be corrected (if possible) or removed. When the outlier is either a legitimate part of the data or the cause is unclear, the issue becomes much more complex. In this case, it is advisable to use robust approaches, in other words, statistical tools designed to produce accurate results even if outliers are present. For a general reference, see Maronna et al. [19], and for a specific reference to robust analysis in neuroimaging data, see Woolrich [20].

Portraying the Distribution of Datasets

Tables are usually the simplest way to present the distribution of a dataset; careful study of them can reveal many characteristics of a dataset. However, "a picture is worth a thousand words," and pictures can be very useful in spotting and revealing structures hidden within the data.

The most common and best understood graphical representation for a continuous outcome is the "histogram," a graphical representation showing a visual impression of the distribution of the observations (see Fig. 3.7 *top panels* for example). Histograms are widely used and familiar, even to nontechnical users, which makes them a convenient way to communicate distributional information to a general audience without the need for extensive explanation. However, as data analysis devices, histograms also have some well-known drawbacks (see Chambers et al. [21]) and, in most cases, it is convenient to also provide additional graphical representation of the data.

"Density plots" are alternatives to histograms (see Fig. 3.7 *bottom plots* for example). They are easily obtained using the formula

$$f(y) = \frac{1}{nh} \sum_{i=1}^{n} W\left(\frac{y - y_i}{h}\right)$$

where the function W is a symmetric but not necessarily positive function (called the kernel) that integrates to one, and $h > 0$ is a smoothing parameter (called the bandwidth). The basic idea is that for each observation y_i, all the observations in the interval $(y_i - 0.5h, y_i + 0.5h)$ are considered and weighted according to the function W. The kernel function does not appear critical while the bandwidth h, which controls how local and how smooth the density estimation will be, needs to be chosen appropriately. For a discussion on this issue, see Bowman and Azzalini [22]. However, all major software implements algorithms for accurate estimation of this tuning parameter without (almost) any intervention from the final user.

"Box-and-whisker plots" (usually referred to simply as boxplots) are becoming increasingly popular for delivering summary displays of the distribution of a dataset (see Fig. 3.8, *center panels* for example). In a boxplot, the lower and upper quartiles of the dataset are depicted by the top and the bottom of a rectangle (the box). The median, which measures the location of the distribution, is depicted as a horizontal segment within the rectangle. Two segments (the whiskers) are portrayed from the end of the box to the Tukey fences. Data values outside the Tukey fences are plotted as individual points. In a boxplot, one can read the most important information on the structure of the data distribution. Location is measured by the position of the median; the spread of the bulk of the data is measured by the length of the box (which includes the central 50 % of the observations); the length of the whiskers gives information on how stretched the tails of the distribution are; the individual outside values evidence observations that appear unusually large or small. If the distribution of the data distribution is symmetric, then the boxplot is symmetric about the median (i.e., the median cuts the box in half), the whisker segments are about the same length, and the outside values at top and bottom (if any) are about equal in number and symmetrically placed. Boxplots are very effective for comparing the distribution of two or more samples. By producing the plots on the same scale, we are able to make direct comparison of the location (medians), interquartile range (spread), and shape. The width of the rectangle usually has no meaning; however, in some cases, it can be used to illustrate the size of each dataset by making the width of the box proportional to the size of the group; a popular convention is to make the box width proportional to the square root of the size of the group.

"Notched boxplots" apply narrowing of the box around the median (see Fig. 3.8, *bottom*

panels for example). The notches extend to $\pm 1.57(Q_3 - Q_1)\big/\sqrt{n}$ (where n denotes the sample size) and offer a rough guide to the significance of the medians: if the notches of two boxes do not overlap, there is evidence of a statistically significant difference between the medians (McGill et al. [23]). The comparison of medians using notched boxplots can be regarded as the graphical analogue (quick and dirty) of a two-sample t-test and one-way analysis of variance.

Tukey [24] also proposed "stem-and-leaf" diagrams (see Fig. 3.7 *center panels* for example). A stem-and-leaf diagram is constructed as two columns separated by a vertical line: the left column contains the "stems" (the leading digits in the range of the data) and the right column contains the "leaves" (trailing digits written in the appropriate row to the right of the line). The plot can be seen as a hybrid between a table and a graph since it shows numerical values as numerals, but its profile is very much like a histogram. This device, which can even be constructed by hand easily, is particularly useful when it is important to convey both numerical values of the observations and graphical information about the distribution. However, stem-and-leaf plots are better suited for moderately sized samples, whereas other devices (boxplots, density trace plots, or even histograms) may become more appropriate for bigger samples.

Empirical "quantile–quantile plots" (QQ-plots) offer a very effective tool for comparison of the distribution of two samples (see Fig. 3.9 for example). As long as the two datasets have the same number of observations, an empirical QQ plot is simply a plot of one sorted dataset against another. If the two distributions are identical, all the points will lie exactly on the straight line passing through the origin with a unit slope. QQ plots offer much more detailed information than a simple comparison of means or medians, since the whole distribution is considered. Nevertheless, this comes at a cost, since we need much more observations than for comparisons based on simple statistical indexes (see Chambers et al. [21]).

Data Modeling

The Normal Probability Model

One of the most useful and frequently encountered models for continuous outcomes is the "normal" (Gaussian) distribution. It plays an important role in statistical analysis, since it can be shown that many real phenomena are very well approximated by a normal distribution (see Fig. 3.1, *left panel*). The formula for the normal probability distribution is given by

$$f(x) = \frac{1}{\sqrt{2\pi\sigma^2}} e^{-\frac{1}{2\sigma^2}(x-\mu)^2}$$

where μ and σ^2 denotes, respectively, the mean and the variance of the variable X, with $\pi \cong 3.1416$ and $e \cong 2.7183$. The normal distribution is unimodal and symmetric about its mean, with spread measured by the value of its variance (or its standard deviation). In Fig. 3.1 (*right panel*), several graphs for normal distribution with different values for μ and σ^2 are depicted. It is clear that curves with greater variance (or standard deviation) denote greater dispersion around the mean, whereas increasing the mean moves the curve along the x axis.

Probabilities are obtained as areas over intervals under the curve of the normal probability distribution (see Fig. 3.2, *left panel*) and are easily computed by referring to some statistical software or to the tabulated probabilities of the standard normal distribution. The latter is obtained from a normal distribution using the transformation $z = (x - \mu)/\sigma$. So, the standard

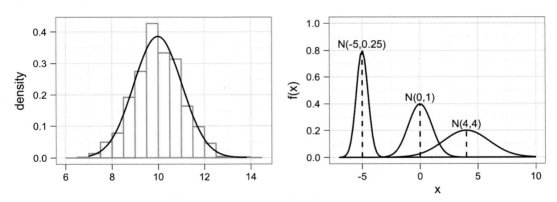

Fig. 3.1 Histogram of a dataset with its normal approximation (*left panel*); several normal distributions with different means and variances (*right panel*)

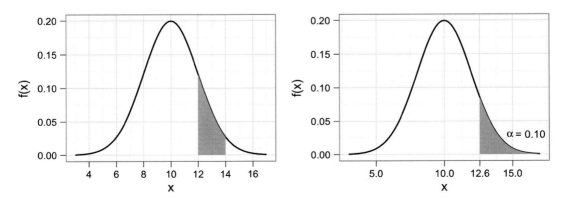

Fig. 3.2 Probability of being inside the interval [12, 14] on a Gaussian distribution with mean equal to 10 and variance equal to 2 (*left panel*); percentile of order 10 % (the value that leaves 10 % of the area at its right) (*right panel*)

normal distribution has $\mu = 0$ and $\sigma^2 = 1$. Figure 3.2 (*right panel*) also depicts the percentile of order $\alpha = 0.10$ as the value that leaves 10 % of the area under the curve at its right. Consequently, all the area under the curve being equal to one, it leaves 90 % of the area at its left.

Assessing Normality

Many statistical procedures rely on the assumption that the observed data are sampled from a Gaussian population. Consequently, there exists a vast literature, including both graphical tools and inferential procedures, for testing whether the normality assumption is reasonable for the data at hand.

An effective graphical tool to assess normality and departure from normality is the "normal probability plot," which compares the quantiles of the observed dataset with those of the Gaussian distribution. A quantile of order α (with $0 \le \alpha \le 1$) of a dataset is a number on the scale of the data that divides it into two groups, so that a fraction α of the observations fall below and a fraction $1 - \alpha$ fall above. For example, a quantile of order 0.80 means that 80 % of the observations fall below the quantile and 20 % fall above the quantile. More formally, given a set of values $y_1, y_2, \cdots, y_n$, sort the values in ascending order $y_{(1)}, y_{(2)}, \cdots, y_{(n)}$. The values $y_{(1)}, y_{(2)}, \cdots, y_{(n)}$ are called the order statistics of the original sample. Take the order statistics to be the quantiles which correspond to the fractions:
$$p_i = (i - 1)\big/(n - 1), \quad \text{for}$$
$i = 1, \cdots, n$. In general, to define the quantile that corresponds to the fraction α, linear interpolation between the two nearest p_i can be used. If α lies a fraction f of the way from p_i to p_{i-1}, define the α quantile to be

$$Q(\alpha) = (1 - f)Q(p_i) + fQ(p_{i-1})$$

The function Q defined in this way is known as the quantile function. Clearly, the median is obtained as $Q(0.50)$, the lower quartile as $Q(0.25)$, and the upper quartile as $Q(0.75)$.

A normal probability plot is constructed by plotting the quantiles of the empirical distribution against the corresponding percentile of the Gaussian distribution (see Fig. 3.10 for example). If the two distributions match, the points on the plot will form a linear pattern passing through the origin with a unit slope. Departures from normality (heavy tails, asymmetry, outliers, mixed distributions, etc.) are reflected as deviation of the points from the linear pattern.

Obviously, a graphical tool can give only some hints about departures from normality. To determine whether or not a dataset is modeled effectively by a normal distribution, normality tests should be used. This type of test verifies the null hypothesis that a sample of observations comes from a normal distribution. Maybe the simplest and most commonly used omnibus test for gaussianity is the Jarque–Bera (JB) test. It is defined as

$$JB = n\left\{\frac{sk}{6} + \frac{(kurt - 3)^2}{24}\right\}$$

where sk is an estimate of the asymmetry of the distribution of the data (in a Gaussian distribution, which is symmetric, this value is expected to be close to zero) and $kurt$ is an estimate of the kurtosis of the data (in a Gaussian distribution, it is expected to be close to 3). Thus, the test statistics use skewness and kurtosis to quantify how far from normality the distribution of the data at hand is, in terms of asymmetry and shape. Increasing values of the test statistics denote more severe departure from the normality assumption. If the null hypothesis is true, the JB test statistic is distributed, approximately, as a chi-squared distribution with 2 degrees of freedom. Therefore, the corresponding p-value can be computed as the probability of obtaining a test statistic at least as extreme as the one that was actually observed, assuming that the null hypothesis is true (i.e., assuming that data have been generated by a Gaussian distribution). The null hypothesis is rejected when p-values are "small," usually when they are less than the significance level α (usually chosen as equal to 0.05 or 0.01). When the null hypothesis is rejected, the result is said to be statistically significant at the level α. In Fig. 3.3, two examples of p-values computed on a chi-squared distribution with 2 degrees of freedom are depicted. In the right panel, the p-value

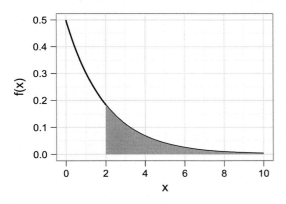
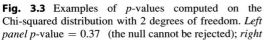
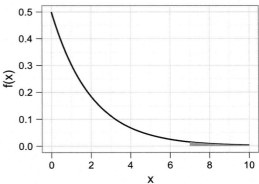

Fig. 3.3 Examples of *p*-values computed on the Chi-squared distribution with 2 degrees of freedom. *Left panel p*-value $= 0.37$ (the null cannot be rejected); *right*

panel p-value $= 0.03$, the null can be rejected at the 0.05 level, but it cannot be rejected at the 0.01 level

is equal to 0.03, so the null can be rejected at the level of 0.05 (the test is statistically significant at the level 0.05). Note that the null cannot be rejected at the level 0.01 (the test is not statistically significant at the level 0.01). In the left panel, the *p*-value is equal to 0.37, so the null cannot be rejected.

As a further remark, please note that in no way does the *p*-value measure the probability of the null hypothesis being true. On the contrary, *p*-values are computed assuming as a condition that the null hypothesis is true.

The JB test is a versatile and powerful (compared with some others) normality test and is often recommended in the literature (Yazici and Yolacan [25]). Other popular choices are the Shapiro–Wilk normality test, the D'Agostino test, the Anderson–Darling test, the Cramér–von-Mises criterion, the Lilliefors test for normality (an adaptation of the Kolmogorov–Smirnov test), and the Shapiro–Francia test for normality, to mention only a few. The Kolmogorov–Smirnov test used to be very popular, but the most recent alternatives appear to be more powerful (i.e., they are more capable of rejecting the normality hypothesis when data come from a distribution that is not Gaussian). For a deeper insight into the huge literature on this topic, see also Thode [26] and the references therein.

As a final remark, please also note that using normality tests could appear to be an easy way to decide whether a parametric or a non-parametric statistical test should be used. However, this is not the case, because the size of the samples used in such tests plays an important role. For very small samples, normality tests are not very useful since they have little power to discriminate between Gaussian and non-Gaussian populations. Small samples simply do not contain enough information for inferences about the shape of the distribution of the entire population. On the other hand, for very large sample sizes, the tests will reject the null even for very mild departures from normality. An interesting comparison and some useful recommendations can be found in Yazici and Yolacan [25].

If the null hypothesis that the sample of observations at hand comes from a normal distribution is not rejected, all statistical tools that require the normality assumption can be safely used. Conversely, if the null is rejected, these tools might lead to biased results and inaccurate conclusions. A possible strategy to deal with this issue is to use some mathematical modification of the original data to achieve a distribution that is as close as possible to a Gaussian shape. For positive data values, in some cases, just taking some simple transformation of the variable (such as the logarithm or the square root) might deliver a distribution that is much closer to the normal. A more general transformation (which includes the logarithmic and the square root as particular cases) is the Box–Cox transformation, which accommodates a whole range of power transformations, available to improve the efficacy of normalizing for both positively and negatively skewed variables (Osborne [27]).

Nevertheless, please note that while data transformations are important options for practitioners, they do fundamentally change the nature of the variable, making the interpretation of the results much more difficult. An alternative approach is to use statistical tools that do not rely on the normality assumption (indeed, they do not require any parametric assumption) and consequently have a much wider field of application. These methods, known as nonparametric methods, are briefly discussed for some applications in the following sections. A very nice review of nonparametrics can be found in Lehmann [28].

Inference from a Single Dataset

One of the most important issues in making inferences from a single dataset is estimation of the location of a given variable measured on a well-defined population. Suppose we are interested in estimating the population mean (α) of some numerical variable of interest Y. This can be achieved by using the random sample drawn from the population of interest and by using the information contained in the sample to learn about the population. Let $y_1, y_2, \cdots, y_n$ be an observed sample of size n from the variable Y. A "point estimate" of the true (unknown) mean μ is simply given by the sample mean $\bar{y}$, in other words the mean of the observations contained in the sample. Clearly, due to sampling variability, the sample mean is unlikely to be exactly equal to the population mean μ: different samples lead to different point estimates. Therefore, to avoid misleading inferences, an accurate estimate of the uncertainty associated with the estimation process based on the observed sample is crucial.

The accuracy of the inference process can be evaluated by looking at the "sampling distribution" of the sample mean. To understand this important concept, imagine collecting all possible samples of size n from the population under study and calculating the sample mean for each of them. The sampling distribution is just the distribution of these mean values. It can be shown that (1) the mean of the sampling distribution of the sample mean (that is the mean of all point estimates based on the sample mean) is equal to the (unknown) population mean; (2) the standard deviation of the sampling distribution (called the "standard error" of the sample mean) is equal to $\sigma / \sqrt{n}$, where σ denotes the population standard deviation. The standard error measures the accuracy of the sample mean in estimating the population mean. The accuracy depends on the variability of the variable Y and on the sample size n: (1) the larger the variability of the population, the lower the estimating accuracy; (2) the larger the sample size, the greater the estimating accuracy. While we seldom know σ we can estimate it by using the sample standard deviation s and get an estimated standard error as $s / \sqrt{n}$. Note that the standard deviation and the standard error should never be confused. The standard deviation (σ) measures the amount of variability in the population (it is not related to the observed sample), whereas the standard error ($\sigma / \sqrt{n}$) measures the accuracy of the sample mean as an estimate of the population parameter μ.

As already discussed in the previous section, using the mean as a measure of location appears to be questionable if the sample includes outlying observations. In this case, some practitioners use what at first sight appears to be a natural strategy: (1) check for extreme values; (2) remove them; (3) compute the sample mean with the remaining data. We advocate against this procedure of discarding outliers and continuing to use the sample mean. Indeed, it can be shown that when outliers are removed, the remaining values are no longer independent; consequently, special techniques are required when estimating the standard error of this peculiar sample mean.

To avoid this practice, when outliers might be present, it is advisable to use the sample median, which provides an important and useful alternative for robust estimation of the location of the population distribution. Indeed, when a distribution is approximately symmetric and no outliers are present in the data, the mean and median estimate—approximately—the same quantity. The sample median can be estimated as follows: (1) sort the observed data in ascending order, to obtain the order statistics $y_{(1)}, y_{(2)}, \cdots, y_{(n)}$; (2) if the sample size n is odd, estimate the median as $Me = y_{((n+1)/2)}$; if n is even, estimate the median as $Me = \left(y_{(n/2)} + y_{(n/2+1)} \right) \Big/ 2$. The standard error of the sample median can be estimated as $\left(y_{(U_n)} - y_{(L_n+1)} \right) \Big/ 2$, where $U_n = n - L_n$ and $L_n = n\big/2 - \sqrt{n\big/4}$ with the operator x denoting the smallest integer $\geq x$ (e.g., $5.3 = 6$) (Olive [29]).

Information about uncertainty measured by the standard error and point estimation can be summarized by a confidence interval for the parameter of interest, the population mean or the population median. A confidence interval for the mean (median) is an interval (i.e., a range of values) that is claimed to include the true population mean (median) with a specified (high) confidence level.

To discuss confidence intervals, it is necessary to introduce a new probability model derived from the Gaussian distribution: the Student's t-distribution. Like the Gaussian, this distribution is symmetric about its mean (which is equal to zero) and is bell shaped. With respect to the Gaussian, the Student's t-distribution has heavier tails, meaning it is more prone to generate values that fall far from its mean. Consequently, for a given percentile, there is a greater tail probability in the Student's t-distribution with respect to the Gaussian (see Fig. 3.4, *right panel*). This makes the t distribution an appropriate model for the statistical behavior of certain types of ratios of random quantities. The exact shape of the t distribution depends on the degrees of freedom: the fewer the degrees of freedom, the heavier the tails of the distribution (see Fig. 3.4, *left panel*). However, the Student's t-distribution converges to the Gaussian distribution when the degrees of freedom increase. For values >30, the two distributions are very similar to each other; for very large values, they are almost indistinguishable.

Confidence Intervals for the Population Mean

Let us assume that the observed data are sampled from a Gaussian distribution. Let $t_{\left(n-1,\frac{\alpha}{2}\right)}$ denote the percentile of order $\alpha/2$ of a Student's t-distribution with $n-1$ degrees of freedom and let $l_{\inf} = \bar{y} - t_{\left(n-1,\frac{\alpha}{2}\right)}\frac{s}{\sqrt{n}}$ and $l_{\sup} = \bar{y} + t_{\left(n-1,\frac{\alpha}{2}\right)}\frac{s}{\sqrt{n}}$. It can be shown that the population mean μ is contained in the interval $[l_{\inf}, l_{\sup}]$ with a confidence level equal to $1 - \alpha$. In other words, if we were to draw

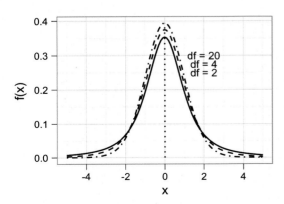
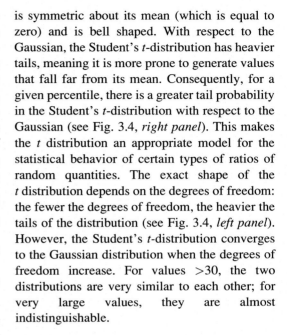
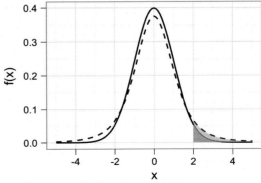

Fig. 3.4 Density function of Student's t-distributions with different degrees of freedom (*left panel*); area under the standard normal curve (*solid line*) and under a Student's t-distribution with 4 degrees of freedom (*dashed line*) for values of x greater than 2; the two areas are respectively equal to 0.0228 and 0.0581 (*right panel*)

all the independent random samples of size n from the population under study, and calculate the corresponding confidence intervals for each sample, we can expect that $100(1 - \alpha)\%$ of these confidence intervals would contain the true population mean, while α % of them would not. For instance, if we fix the confidence level $(1 - \alpha)$ equal to 0.95, this means we expect the corresponding interval will not include the true population values 5 % of the time. The confidence level can also be fixed equal to 0.90 or 0.99 to reduce or increase, respectively, the confidence of covering the true parameter value.

Clearly, the shorter the length of the confidence interval, the more accurate the estimation of the population mean. The confidence interval length is a function of (1) the confidence level (the higher the confidence level, the longer the confidence interval); (2) the population variability (the higher the population variability, the higher the standard error estimate and the longer the confidence interval); (3) the sample size (the higher the sample size, the lower the standard error and the shorter the confidence interval). Please note that the sample size in the standard error formula is under the square root sign, which means that if one wishes to halve the confidence interval length, it is not sufficient to double the sample size (keeping fixed all other values).

If the sample size is large enough, the Student's t-distribution can be safely approximated by the standard normal distribution (the greater the sample size, the better the approximation). In this case, the confidence limits of a $100(1 - \alpha)\%$ of an approximate confidence interval for the mean can be computed as $l_{\inf} = \bar{y} - z_{\frac{\alpha}{2}}\frac{s}{\sqrt{n}}$ and $l_{\sup} = \bar{y} + z_{\frac{\alpha}{2}}\frac{s}{\sqrt{n}}$, where $z_{\frac{\alpha}{2}}$ denotes the percentile of order $\alpha/2$ of the standard normal distribution.

If the data are sampled from a non-Gaussian distribution, an approximate confidence interval for the population mean can still be computed as before. Again, accuracy increases with sample size. However, there is no general rule to establish what a "large" sample is. Some recent studies show there are general conditions that lead to

sample sizes much larger than previously thought for acceptable results (see Wilcox [5] for a discussion on this point).

Confidence Intervals for the Population Median

A similar approach can be used to construct a confidence interval for the population median. A $100(1 - \alpha)\%$ confidence interval for the median is given by $[l_{\inf}, l_{\sup}]$, where

$$l_{\inf} = Me - t_{\left(g, \frac{\alpha}{2}\right)}\left(y_{(U_n)} - y_{(L_n+1)}\right)/2 \quad \text{and}$$

$$l_{\sup} = Me + t_{\left(g, \frac{\alpha}{2}\right)}\left(y_{(U_n)} - y_{(L_n+1)}\right)/2 \quad \text{with}$$

$g = U_n - L_n - 1$ (see Olive [29]).

Again, for "large" samples, the confidence intervals for the median can be calibrated using the standard normal percentiles instead of those of the Student's t-distribution (i.e., it is possible to use $z_{\frac{\alpha}{2}}$ instead of $t_{\left(g, \frac{\alpha}{2}\right)}$).

It is important to stress that using the mean and the median is not a case of "one or the other" as computation of confidence intervals for both cases can deliver invaluable numerical information to identify situations where observed data deserve deeper insights. Understanding why the classical confidence interval for the mean is substantially different from that for the median can be very informative. Under the usual assumptions of approximate normality (which also implies distributional symmetry), the mean and the median should be very close to each other. If this is not the case, these assumptions might have been violated because of outliers, marked distributional asymmetry, or other less common departures from normality.

So far, we have shown that confidence intervals can be easily constructed using the sampling distribution of the estimate of the parameter of interest: the population mean or the population median. This sampling distribution is either known (e.g., a Student's t-distribution) or can be approximated by the normal distribution if the sample is large enough. In this latter case, the standard normal distribution is used to compute the percentiles for a given level of confidence, which in turn are necessary to compute the limits of the confidence intervals. In general, this approach can deliver acceptable results but, in many practical situations and for small and moderate sample sizes, approximating the sampling distribution of interest by using the normal distribution can be highly unsatisfactory (see Wilcox [5] for a discussion on this point). This appears to be evident from Fig. 3.5. For data sampled from a Gaussian distribution, the Student's t-distribution is the exact sampling distribution of the studentized sample mean (left panel), and confidence intervals constructed using this distribution are very accurate. However, for data sampled from an asymmetric distribution, the Student's t is not a good approximation of the true sampling distribution, which is markedly asymmetric with large differences in the tails (right panel). This implies that the percentiles computed using the Student's t-distribution are wrong and confidence intervals based on them will no longer be accurate.

One of the many alternative strategies available to overcome these problems is to use bootstrap confidence intervals.

Confidence Intervals Based on the Bootstrap

Bootstrapping is a general statistical technique, the implementation of which is based on a very simple yet powerful principle: many repeated samples are drawn from the original sample, and inference is made from those samples

(Efron [30]). The name derives from the expression "pulling oneself up by one's bootstraps," and it is intended to stress that no additional data or strong parametric assumptions on the underlying population are needed to make inference. The bootstrap is a computer-intensive technique that (1) allows the researcher to construct inference procedures without assuming normality or symmetry (which are difficult to verify in small samples) and (2) can deliver more accurate results than the standard normal approximation, under quite general conditions.

The bootstrap algorithm to estimate the sampling distribution of the sample mean runs as follows:

1. From the original dataset $y_1, y_2, \cdots, y_n$ draw with replacement a sample of size n to obtain a bootstrap dataset, $y_1^*, y_2^*, \cdots, y_n^*$.
2. Calculate the bootstrap version of the sample mean, that is, compute $\bar{y}^* = \left(1/n\right) \sum_{i=1}^{n} y_i^*$.
3. Repeat steps (1) and (2) several times, say B times, obtaining B bootstrap estimates of the mean $\bar{y}_1^*, \bar{y}_2^*, \cdots, \bar{y}_B^*$.
4. Use the empirical distribution of these B bootstrap estimates (i.e., the collection of values obtained from the bootstrap process) as an approximation of the sampling distribution of the statistics of interest. This bootstrap distribution can be used to estimate either

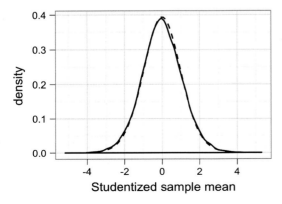
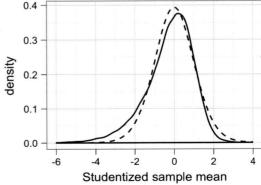

Fig. 3.5 True sampling distribution of the studentized sample mean (sample size $n = 20$) estimated via Monte Carlo simulation (*solid line*) vs. Student's t-distribution with $n - 1 = 19$ degrees of freedom (*dashed line*) for data sampled from a Gaussian distribution (*left panel*) and from an asymmetric distribution (*right panel*)

standard errors or percentiles to be used for the construction of confidence intervals. To compute the bootstrap percentiles, sort the bootstrap estimates into ascending order and estimate percentiles by selecting appropriate order statistics.

The bootstrap approach can deliver accurate inference, even for small sample sizes and for both symmetric and asymmetric distributions. Figure 3.6 depicts the true sampling distribution of the sample mean for a small sample ($n = 20$) along with its bootstrap approximation. In both symmetric (left panel) and asymmetric (right panel) cases, the bootstrap is able to deliver an approximation that is very close to the true unknown sampling distribution.

The bootstrap scheme discussed above can be easily adapted to estimate the sampling distribution of the sample median: along the same algorithm, simply use the sample median in place of the sample mean to obtain the bootstrap replicates of the sample median.

By using the bootstrap, we seek to mimic, in an appropriate manner, the way the sample is collected from the population in the process of bootstrap sampling from the observed data. Note that when resampling with replacement, a data point is randomly selected from the original dataset and copied into the resampled dataset being created. Although that data point has been already "used," it is not deleted from the

original dataset. Another data point is then randomly selected, and the process is repeated until a resampled dataset of size n is created. As a result, the same observation might be included in the resampled dataset one, two, or more times, or not at all.

A key issue when using the bootstrap is fixing the number of bootstrap replicates (B). Basically, this is strictly connected to the nature of the statistical problem one wishes to solve. For 90 % or 95 % confidence intervals, a figure between 1000 and 2000 is usually adequate (see Efron and Tibshirani [31], among others). However, for simple statistics, such as the mean or the median, larger values can be freely fixed, because of the increasing computing power available nowadays, even in standard personal computers. Additionally, B should also be fixed such that $(1 - \alpha)(B + 1)$ is a whole number. This implies that for the common choices of the confidence level $(1 - \alpha)$, most practitioners choose $B = 999$ or $B = 1999$. This allows simpler process for selection of order statistics and less biased percentile estimation (Hall [32]).

The bootstrap can be used for many statistical purposes, yet one of the most common is to compute confidence intervals. The simplest bootstrap confidence interval is the "bootstrap percentile confidence interval": for a confidence level equal to $(1 - \alpha)$, it is simply defined as the range within which $100(1 - \alpha)\%$ of bootstrapped statistics fall. For example, to

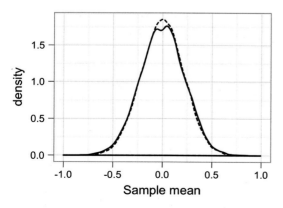
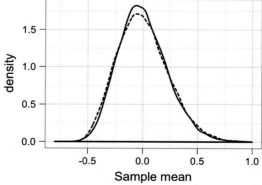
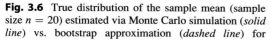

Fig. 3.6 True distribution of the sample mean (sample size $n = 20$) estimated via Monte Carlo simulation (*solid line*) vs. bootstrap approximation (*dashed line*) for samples drawn from a Gaussian distribution (*left panel*) and from an asymmetric distribution (*right panel*). The true distributions have zero mean

construct a 95 % confidence interval for the population mean, we simply take the middle 95 % of the bootstrap sample means, using as confidence limits the 0.025 and 0.975 percentiles of the bootstrap distribution.

However, even if this method is easy to apply, more accurate confidence intervals for the population mean can be obtained using the "bootstrap-t method." It runs as follows:

1. From the original dataset $y_1, y_2, \cdots, y_n$, draw with replacement a sample of size n to obtain a bootstrap dataset, $y_1^*, y_2^*, \cdots, y_n^*$.
2. Use the bootstrap samples to compute the quantities $t^* = \sqrt{n}(\bar{y}^* - \bar{y})/s^*$, where $s*$ is the sample variance computed on the bootstrap replicate.
3. Repeat steps (1) and (2) several times, say B times, obtaining B bootstrap estimates of the statistic $t_1^*, t_2^*, \cdots, t_B^*$.
4. Sort the bootstrap values $t_1^*, t_2^*, \cdots, t_B^*$ in ascending order, yielding $t_{(1)}^*, t_{(2)}^*, \cdots, t_{(B)}^*$.
5. Fix the confidence level, say $(1 - \alpha) = 0.95$. Fix $B = 999$ (or $B = 1999$) and compute $L = 0.025(B + 1)$ and $U = 0.975(B + 1)$. Compute the percentiles of order 0.025 and 0.975 as, respectively, $t_{(L)}^*$ and $t_{(U)}^*$.
6. Compute the bootstrap-t confidence interval for μ, as $[l_{\text{inf}}, l_{\text{sup}}]$, where $l_{\text{inf}} = \bar{y} - t_{(U)}^* s/\times \sqrt{n}$ and $l_{\text{sup}} = \bar{y} - t_{(L)}^* s/\sqrt{n}$.

In principle, this approach for bootstrap interval construction could be easily extended to the case of the median. However, care must be used, since not all variations of bootstrap schemes perform well for a given estimation problem. For the median case, the basic bootstrap interval can deliver more accurate results (Carpenter and Bithell [33]). It runs as follows:

1. From the original dataset $y_1, y_2, \cdots, y_n$, draw with replacement a sample of size n to obtain a bootstrap dataset, $y_1^*, y_2^*, \cdots, y_n^*$.
2. Use the bootstrap samples to compute the quantities $w^* = Me^* - Me$, where Me is the

sample median computed on the original sample and Me^* is the sample median computed on the bootstrap sample.
3. Repeat steps (1) and (2) several times, say B times, yielding $w_1^*, w_2^*, \cdots, w_B^*$.
4. Sort the bootstrap values $w_1^*, w_2^*, \cdots, w_B^*$ in ascending order, obtaining $w_{(1)}^*, w_{(2)}^*, \cdots, w_{(B)}^*$.
5. Fix the confidence level, say $(1 - \alpha) = 0.95$. Fix $B = 999$ (or $B = 1999$) and compute $L = 0.025(B + 1)$ and $U = 0.975(B + 1)$. Compute the percentiles of order 0.025 and 0.975 as, respectively, $w_{(L)}^*$ and $w_{(U)}^*$.
6. Compute the basic bootstrap interval for Me, as $[l_{\text{inf}}, l_{\text{sup}}]$, where $l_{\text{inf}} = Me - w_{(U)}^*$ and $l_{\text{sup}} = Me - w_{(L)}^*$.

Under appropriate conditions, better confidence intervals can be obtained by computing and correcting for estimation bias and skewness in the bootstrap distribution. This leads to methods that are accurate in a wide variety of setting, for example, the bias-corrected (BC) method and the bias-corrected and accelerated (BC_a) method (the latter being the preferred option). Details on these approaches can be found in Efron and Tibshirani [31] or in Davidson and Hinkley [34]. However, all bootstrap methods for confidence interval construction have, as usual, both advantages and disadvantages and, under particular assumptions, they can even deliver the same result. Some details and a deeper discussion on this point can be found in Carpenter and Bithell [33].

In Table 3.1, we reported, as an example, 95 % confidence intervals for the population mean of a sample of 20 observations drawn both from a Gaussian distribution and from an asymmetric distribution. In both cases, the true population mean is equal to 1. Confidence intervals have been constructed using both asymptotic approximation and alternative bootstrap methods. For the Gaussian distribution case, the exact confidence interval is available and has also been reported. All methods deliver very similar results for the symmetric case, with

Table 3.1 95 % confidence intervals for the population mean of a Gaussian and asymmetric distribution by using asymptotic approximation and alternative bootstrap methods

Method	Symmetric			Asymmetric		
	CI	Length	Shape	CI	Length	Shape
Exact	(0.395, 1.502)	1.107	1.000	–	–	–
Normal	(0.428, 1.467)	1.039	1.000	(0.691, 1.481)	0.790	1.000
Basic	(0.430, 1.468)	1.038	1.001	(0.671, 1.453)	0.782	0.891
t-Bootstrap	(0.391, 1.528)	1.137	1.039	(0.720, 1.683)	0.963	1.164
Percentile	(0.430, 1.467)	1.037	0.999	(0.716, 1.499)	0.783	1.124
BCa	(0.437, 1.476)	1.039	1.031	(0.75, 1.572)	0.820	1.466

For the Gaussian distribution, the exact confidence interval is also available and reported. In both cases, the true population mean is equal to 1

the bootstrap-t method giving a confidence interval very close to the exact one. The confidence interval length (measured as $l_{\text{sup}} - l_{\text{inf}}$) is basically comparable, and the shape (measured as $\left(l_{\text{sup}} - \bar{x}\right) \big/ (\bar{x} - l_{\text{inf}})$) is equal to 1 for the exact and the normal approximation cases (denoting a perfect symmetric interval about the sample mean). Shapes are also very close to 1 for the bootstrap intervals.

On the other hand, for the asymmetric case, results appear to be more variable, in terms of both length and shape. In particular, for all bootstrap intervals the shape is not equal to one, denoting asymmetric confidence intervals about the mean (correctly reflecting the asymmetric nature of the population distribution). This characteristic is clearly missed by the confidence interval obtained using the normal approximation, which is instead symmetric.

Closing this section, a final remark applies. In many statistical applications, the problem is not stated as an estimation problem but instead as a testing problem: the researcher is interested in verifying whether the data provide any evidence that the population mean is equal to a given known value. In other words, the researcher wishes to test the null hypothesis $H_0 : \mu = \mu_0$, where μ_0 is a known value. However, this can be easily achieved by exploiting an interesting relationship between confidence intervals and hypothesis testing. Given a $(1 - \alpha)\%$ confidence interval, if it includes the unknown value μ_0, the null cannot be rejected; otherwise the null can be rejected at the level α. The size of the test α is also the probability of incorrectly rejecting the null hypothesis. A similar construction can be derived for testing the median of the population.

Comparing Two Datasets

In biomedical applications, it is usually of great interest to compare the outcomes of two groups, one including individuals exposed to a risk factor (treatment group) and the other including unexposed individuals (control group). In this framework, two problems are usually addressed: (1) What does the difference between the sample means in the two groups tell us about the difference between the two population means? (2) Do the data provide any evidence that the treatment really affects the outcome variable? Or, on the other hand, has the observed difference in the sample means arisen by chance (solely as a consequence of sampling variability)?

The first problem can be addressed by calculating a confidence interval for the difference of the two population means, following an approach similar to that described in the previous section, to analyze a single dataset.

The second problem can be addressed by hypothesis testing, in other words by looking for empirical evidence against the null hypothesis that there is no difference between the two groups. Evidence is gathered by collecting relevant data and assessing their consistency with the null hypothesis as measured by a *p*-value, which is defined as the probability of recording a difference between the two groups at least as large as that of the dataset at hand (if there were no effect of the treatment in the population).

Specifically, when comparing two populations, the null hypothesis of no difference between the two population means can be formally written as $H_0 : \mu_1 = \mu_2$, where μ_1 denotes the mean of the first population (control group) and μ_2 the population mean of the second population (treatment group). To check this hypothesis, it is very important to discern between the case in which the data are paired and that in which the groups are independent.

Paired data arise when two outcomes are measured on the same individual under different treatment circumstances. Alternatively, pairs may also be obtained when considering groups of different individuals who are matched during sample selection as they share certain key characteristics such as sex, age, etc. In this case, the sample is made of pairs of observations, each pair made of data values recorded for a single individual in two different circumstances. Let $d_1, d_2, \cdots, d_n$ be the sample differences measured on each individual and let $t = \overline{d}\big/\mathrm{SE}$ $\left(\overline{d}\right)$ be the observed value of the statistic used for testing the null hypothesis, where $\overline{d}$ is the sample mean of the observed differences and $\mathrm{SE}\left(\overline{d}\right)$ is its standard error. To check if this observed sample value is consistent with the null hypothesis of no difference between the two population means, we can compute the corresponding p-value, that is, the probability of getting a difference at least as big as that observed in the sample, if the null is true. Assuming the null distribution is true, if data are drawn from a Gaussian population, this probability can be computed using a Student's t-distribution with $n-1$ degrees of freedom. Small values for the p-value give evidence against the null. For example, if the observed value of the test statistic is $t = 3.1$, the corresponding p-value is equal to 0.012. This means that if the null hypothesis is correct, the probability of observing a difference at least as extreme as 3.1 is equal to 1.2 %. In other words, in the case in which the

null were true, if we extracted all the samples of size n from the target population, we could expect such a large difference in only 1.2 % of cases. The lower the p-value, the stronger the evidence against the null hypothesis. Usually, p-values <5 % are assumed as giving sufficient evidence against the null. As in the previous section, if the sample size is large, the Student's t-distribution can be approximated by the standard Gaussian distribution.

If observations are not paired but are the result of random sampling from two independent populations, testing the null $H_0 : \mu_1 = \mu_2$ should follow different testing schemes. If we can assume that both populations have a Gaussian distribution and also that the variances of the two populations are the same, we can use as test statistics $t = (\overline{x}_2 - \overline{x}_1)\big/SE(\overline{x}_2 - \overline{x}_1)$, where $\overline{x}_2$ and $\overline{x}_1$ are the sample mean of the treatment and of the control group. The standard error of the sample mean difference can be computed as

$$\mathrm{SE}(\overline{x}_2 - \overline{x}_1) = s\sqrt{1\big/n_2 + 1\big/n_1},\ \text{where}$$

$$s^2 = \frac{(n_2 - 1)s_2^2 + (n_1 - 1)s_1^2}{n_2 + n_1 - 2}$$

and $s_2{}^2$ and $s_1{}^2$ are the sample variances of the of the treatment and of the control group, and n_2 and n_1 are the two sample sizes (which do not need to be the same). Under the assumption that the null distribution is true, the p-value can be computed using a Student t-distribution with $n_2 + n_1 - 2$ degrees of freedom.

If the assumption of normality is reasonable, but the variability of the two populations cannot be assumed to be equal, the previous test might deliver inaccurate results. Even if the t-test is known to be robust to "mild" departures from the assumptions, it is difficult to say how different the variances can be before we cannot use the t-test. However, for large samples, even for unequal variances, it is possible to use the normal approximation to compute p-values. In this latter case, the standard error can be more easily computed as $\mathrm{SE}(\overline{x}_2 - \overline{x}_1) = \sqrt{s_2^2\big/n_2 + s_2^2\big/n_1}$.

For small samples, for Gaussian distributions with unequal variances, it is better to use the Welch test, which allows for unequal variances (see Armitage and Berry [35], among others).

If the normality assumption is not reasonable, the t-test might still deliver accurate results for large samples. Alternatively, it is possible to compare the two groups using nonparametric tools as a substitute of the t test. For paired data, it is possible to use the Wilcoxon matched pairs signed rank sum test; for independent groups, it is possible to use the Mann–Whitney test. Both the tests are based on the ranks of the observations and thus use more information than equivalent tests based only on medians. Space constraints mean we only briefly discuss the Mann–Whitney test here. A detailed review on nonparametric tests can be found in Altman [1] or in Wayne [3], whereas a much more technical description can be found in Lehmann [28] or in Hollander and Wolfe [36].

The Mann–Whitney test runs as follows: (1) rank all the observations from both groups together in ascending order of magnitude (if any of these values are equal, average their ranks); (2) sum all the ranks of the observations in the smaller group (either group can be taken if they are of the same size) and denote this sum as "T"; (3) for small samples, compute p-values using appropriate tables (see Altman [1]) or some statistical software; for large samples (ten or more in each group), approximate the sampling distribution of the test statistic T with a Gaussian distribution with mean $\mu_T = n_S(n_S + n_L + 1)\big/2$ (S denoting the smaller group and L the larger one) and variance $\sigma_T^2 = n_L\,\mu_T\big/6$. So, the value of the normalized test statistics $z_T = (T - \mu_T)\big/\sigma_T$ can be used to compute the p-value of the test using the Gaussian distribution

The Mann–Whitney test, while a nonparametric test, still needs to fulfill appropriate assumptions to deliver accurate results: (1) the two samples have been independently and randomly drawn from their respective populations; (2) the variable of interest is continuous; (3) if the populations differ at all, they differ only with respect to their medians. This latter condition is particularly important for the interpretation of the results. If it is fulfilled, the test actually compares the medians of the two populations, and rejecting the null means rejecting the hypothesis that the two medians are equal. However, in practical applications, differences in population medians are often accompanied by differences in the distributions as a whole (spread and shape differences, to mention the most important). So, rejection of the null in the Mann–Whitney test can also be obtained when medians are comparable, but there are significant differences in the spread or in the shape of the two distributions. Thus, the rejection of the null in the Mann–Whitney test requires a deeper analysis of the distribution of the two datasets, and delivering only the p-value of this test can be insufficient and questionable. Conversely, it is very important to look at general distributional differences with a clear discussion about the features that are most important for the data analysis at hand (see Hart [37]). Finally, please note that the Mann–Whitney test as described is based on the assumption that there are no tied ranks. If there are many tied values, some (complicated) corrections need to be applied (for a technical discussion, see Lehman [28]). However, most software packages already account for these corrections, making them readily available for practitioners.

If the t-test rejects the null that the mean of the two populations are equal, it is of interest to estimate this difference by constructing a proper confidence interval. If we deal with paired observations, confidence intervals for the mean difference in the two populations can easily be constructed using all the techniques described in the previous section. Indeed, the test statistic in this case is obtained by turning the sample of pairs of observations into a single sample of differences. Consequently, confidence intervals can be computed using this single dataset. Knowing the standard error and the reference distribution (a Student's t- or a Gaussian distribution) makes it easy to also construct confidence intervals for the difference between the mean of two independent populations. Space constraints prevent discussion of these techniques, but details can be found in Altman [1] or in Wayne

[3]. For the nonparametric case, one can use the bootstrap (see Shao and Tu [38]) or some statistics based on ranks (Bauer [39]).

Software

Many software packages with a range of different characteristics and proprieties and covering a broad spectrum of applications are available for statistical analysis. This section is not intended to be comprehensive or a technical comparison of the software, as this would be largely out of the scope of this chapter. Furthermore, any comparison should be designed with specific fields of application in mind and should look at specific statistical tools. Good general statistical software can often be weak in specific fields where specialized software can excel. Thus, a complete list of all statistical tools, including those available for specific tasks, would require a specific review process and will not be addressed here. Nevertheless, when possible, we report references for an overview and comparison of some software, so the reader can judge how close each piece of software is to his/her needs.

When looking at statistical software, the first distinction is between "closed" products and statistical programming languages. In "closed" statistical software, the user can only perform menu operations alongside the options programmed by the software house. This approach simplifies access to statistical tools (especially if the graphical user interface [GUI] is well designed) for non-experts and practitioners; however, it does not allow the user to program any arbitrarily complex sequence of statistical analysis operations if needed. To accommodate this, most modern statistical software is designed to provide both an environment for statistical and graphical operations and some kind of scripting language that allows automation of repetitive tasks.

The second distinction is between general and specialized software. Some statistical software is general purpose and covers a wide range of applications. Clearly, this wide audience target usually prevents software houses from implementing all the specific features and details that can be found in smaller specialized software.

Moreover, even general-purpose software has its own strengths and weaknesses and so are better suited for application in specific fields.

The third distinction is between commercial and open-source/free software. Some of the software we mention is designed and sold by large companies that can provide high-level support, both on the product itself and on the most effective solutions for specific problems customers may have. Obviously, this comes at a cost that should be carefully evaluated. Use of this type of software for statistical analysis usually requires thorough planning that also involves training of human resources to use the software to its full potential. On the other hand, free software is by no means bad software or without support facilities. Some open-source statistical software is developed at a professional level and used by such a large community that technical support can also be fast and accurate. However, free statistical software does not necessarily mean no cost at all; some level of user training is always necessary. Moreover, most commercial statistical software grants substantial discounts for academic or non-profit use.

Therefore, the choice of statistical software depends on several conditions. First, what budget is available? Some statistical software is very expensive, others are cheaper and some are completely free. Second, what human resources are available? Some software entails a very steep learning curve and specific training to gain the best use, both from a statistical viewpoint and in terms of the software itself; other packages are very user friendly and can be used effectively with a little general training. Finally, what type of statistical analysis is needed? In some cases, some kind of general statistical software is sufficient; in other cases, the required statistical tools are available only in very specific software.

Nevertheless, once these choices are made, plenty of resources are available to assist with getting the best out of the chosen software. For the software reported in this section, it is usually possible to find manuals, books, websites, conferences, journals, and web-based communities of users that can solve almost any problem the user can encounter when using the software.

The most commonly used general-purpose packages in biomedical research are SAS and Statistical Package for the Social Sciences (SPSS).

SAS (Statistical Analysis System) software (developed by the SAS Institute Inc.) is a comprehensive set of integrated tools and solutions for accessing, managing, and analyzing data. SAS is widely used in academic, business, and government organizations, especially when very large databases are to be processed and analyzed. The software comprises a number of separately licensed components to install, which, on one hand, adds great flexibility, allowing the software to be tailored to specific customer needs; however, on the other hand, license costs can quickly increase. The software covers a wide range of statistical applications, including biomedical research as well as forecasting, econometrics, data mining, text mining, and operations research. Statistical analysis in SAS is implemented as SAS programs, a sequence of operations to be performed on data stored as tables. The functionalities of SAS are accessible as statements or procedures via an application–programming interface. A GUI is available, but it should be seen simply as a front end to facilitate the generation of SAS programs. SAS provides power and excellent flexibility. It is ideal for big companies with a large data warehouse, as it runs not only on personal computers with Microsoft® Windows or Linux but also on enterprise-class environments such as Unix, IBM mainframes, and OpenVMS Alpha (SAS programs can be moved almost transparently between these environments). Consequently, it is not intended for casual usage; it requires an appropriate budget and personnel with specific training to exploit its full potential. The learning curve is quite steep and requires some kind of long-term investment in the software. SAS programming is a skill that requires a training period but that also constitutes a professional skill in itself that is useful in the statistics job market. Plenty of resources are available (courses, manuals, books) and a well-organized SAS community exists with user groups on local, regional, and international scales. An overview of SAS software can be found in Rodriguez [40].

IBM SPSS was first released at the end of the 1960s and is now one of the most widely used programs for statistical analysis in social science and related fields. The software (acquired by IBM in 2009) covers a large number of statistical techniques, most of which are accessible with a user-friendly GUI via pull-down menus. The software is easy to learn and use, making statistical analysis available to the casual user. On the other hand, it is convenient for the experienced user since it includes a full range of data management and editing tools, in-depth statistical capabilities, and complete plotting, reporting, and presentation features. Moreover, specific algorithms and complex data manipulation and analyses can be programmed via a proprietary script language, which is also useful for simplifying repetitive tasks. Like SAS, the software consists of a number of separately licensed components to install. Again, this adds great flexibility but can quickly increase costs. SPSS is available on virtually all computing platforms, including Microsoft® Windows, Macintosh, and Linux. Similar to SAS, plenty of resources (courses, manuals, books) and web communities are available for support and insights into using the software.

Both SAS and SPSS are excellent software; however, they might be beyond the budget of some users. Other very good alternative software is available at a lower cost.

Stata is general-purpose statistical software well known for its wide range of statistical routines, ease of data management, and publication-quality graphics. The software appeals to researchers from a wide range of fields and is used by many institutions (both academic and non-academic) around the world, especially in the fields of economics, sociology, political science, biomedicine, and epidemiology. Stata runs on several personal computer operating systems (including Windows, Macintosh, and several Unix/Linux distributions) and can be used by both a command line interface and a point-and-click menu interface, with one-to-one correspondence between the two. As with the previously mentioned software, Stata has its own interpretive language that allows experienced users to program their own routines to implement new algorithms not available in the standard distribution. Stata is offered as a standard version that is appropriate for most purposes (Stata/IC), an expanded version useful with larger datasets (Stata/SE), and a version specifically designed to take advantage of multiple cores/processors that run faster on systems that have them (Stata/MP). Many resources (manuals, courses, books) make Stata accessible to new users. There exists also an active community of Stata users, Stata conferences, and a journal, *The Stata Journal*, that publishes reviewed scientific papers about statistics, data analysis, and effective use of the software. Hilbe [41] and in Gutierrez [42] provide an overview of this software.

STATISTICA (StatSoft) is another general-purpose, comprehensive, and well-designed software that covers a broad range of statistical techniques accessible by a very user friendly GUI that uses ribbon bars much like the last versions of Microsoft® Office. This makes the software easy to learn and use, providing an environment that most user are accustomed to working within. As with other software, repetitive tasks can be programmed using a scripting language, STATISTICA Visual Basic, which includes the general Visual Basic programming environment and the *STATISTICA* libraries to allow access to the statistical functionality of the software. Moreover, STATISTICA integrates well with other software, such as the statistical language R, Microsoft Office, Microsoft OLE DB, or SAP Business Warehouse. For a review of a previous version of the software, see Hilbe [45].

SYSTAT is another general-purpose statistical package designed for statistical analysis and graphical presentation of scientific data. The software provides a wide variety of statistical tools and a range of graphs that is one of the richest among available statistical software. Nevertheless, SYSTAT is characterized by a small footprint (it has smaller RAM and disk space requirements than other statistical packages). The GUI is a strength, and it also has available a scripting language for programming repetitive tasks. The latest version (13.1) appears to be available solely for Microsoft Windows, but the company claims it runs smoothly in Mac OS X using some virtualization software. For an overview of this software, see Wilkinson [47] and Hilbe [42–44].

MedCalc is software specifically designed to help biomedical researchers with statistics analysis. It covers and makes readily available almost all of the statistical tools usually employed in analyzing medical data. It has a very small footprint but runs only on Microsoft Windows. The software is not as rich and complete as the previous examples, but this could also be seen as a strength. It focuses on a subset of techniques useful in medical research that are easily accessible via a GUI, and it is not overwhelming for practitioners with a limited background in statistics.

JMP (SAS Institute Inc.) is another comprehensive statistical package that covers a great number of statistical tools useful to scientists operating in different fields. What makes this software unique is its interactive nature that makes discoveries and learning through data exploration easy and available to users with a limited statistical background. JMP's GUI makes plots interactive, dynamically linking data with graphics for interactive exploration, understanding, and visualization. In other words, in JMP, it is possible to click on any point in a graph and see the corresponding data point highlighted in the data table and in other graphs. This can make discovering hidden structures within the data easy and accessible, even for the casual user. Moreover, in designing JMP's GUI, priority was given to a smooth and natural workflow for data analysis, allowing the user to focus on the problem at hand and not on the technicalities of the software. JMP has a flexible working environment with a user-friendly menu-based interface, but it also allows for custom programming and script development for routine tasks. The software, originally developed for the Macintosh, is now supported by both Mac OS X and Microsoft Windows operating systems (Linux appears unsupported since 2010). Two further JMP products are of great interest for medical researchers and bio-scientists: JMP Clinical (for data discovery, analysis and reporting for clinical trials) and JMP Genomics (for genomics and analysis of microarray data). An overview of this software can be found in Jones and Sall [46].

R is an open-source implementation of the S language, a statistical programming language developed by Bell laboratories during the 1970s. R is both a powerful statistical environment and a flexible programming language that can be used to perform statistical analyses, to manipulate datasets, and to produce high-quality graphics (R Core Team [49]). The functionality of R can be extended by R users (by writing code to implement new procedures), and it has emerged as the primary statistical research tool in statistics and bioinformatics. Additional functionalities to the R language are usually included and delivered in packages, and thousands of packages are currently available that cover both general and very specific statistical applications. R is also free, which may be an attractive feature for those researchers who cannot afford a license for proprietary software or when the software is used in multicore/multiprocessor environments, where commercial software usually charges the license fee as a function of the number of available cores/processors. R is cross platform (it runs on Microsoft Windows, Mac OS X, and GNU/Linux) and is actively supported by thousands of contributors and millions of users, with plenty of free documentation and web resources. Bioconductor is a very active open source and open development project based on R. It provides more than 1000 packages with specific tools for statistical applications to bioscience for the analysis and comprehension of high-throughput genomic data. As a drawback, to exploit all the power of R, data need to be manipulated from the command line, which can appear quite difficult to use, with a steep learning curve, especially compared with statistical environments where data are manipulated via a GUI. In any case, some integrated development environments (IDE) are available for R, such as Rstudio, making the use of R much more accessible to practitioners. Moreover, some GUIs such as R commander or JCR, albeit not as complete

as those available in commercial software, can be used for standard R usage. As an example of the popularity of R language among researchers and practitioners, and how rich the set of statistical tools available in R, both STATISTICA and SPSS—market leaders in commercial statistical software—allow integration with R, making its statistical tools and procedures available within their standard GUI and workflow. Native R scripts can be run directly within STATISTICA, and R output can be retrieved as native STATISTICA spreadsheets and graphs. In the same spirit, SPSS developed the IBM SPSS Statistics Developer, which is a program for wrapping R functions in a format that allows them to run in SPSS. Splus also offers language extensions for R package compatibility.

Spreadsheet software, such as Microsoft Excel, are widespread tools used for quick and easy data management in almost every statistical analysis workflow. This software also offers limited statistical analysis support that covers all basic standard tools, including tables, graphs, summaries, and basic inference procedures (t-tests, analysis of variance [ANOVA], and regression modeling). However, some authors advocate against the use of Excel (and other spreadsheet software) for serious statistical analysis (see McCullogh and Wilson [48,50]; McCullogh and Heiser [51]). In any case, it is possible to exploit the wide penetration of this software in all fields of applied statistics by enhancing its statistical capabilities with add-in packages. These tools have been developed by several software houses to carry out sophisticated and accurate statistical analysis within the comfortable and very well known Excel framework. A comprehensive and very good add-in is XLSTAT, which includes both basic and advanced tools for statistical analysis; however, several other alternatives are available and can also be considered: StatEL, Analyse-it, WinSTAT, StatTools, UNISTAT.

Examples

The dataset considered for these examples is the Echocardiogram dataset from the UCI Machine Learning Repository (Frank and Asuncion [52]).

The sample is made of 13 variables observed in 132 patients. All the patients had experienced heart attacks at some point in the past. Some have survived; others have not. The "survival" and "still-alive" variables, when taken together, indicate whether a patient survived for at least 1 year following the heart attack.

Figure 3.7 depicts histograms (*two top panels*), stem-and-leaf plots (*central panels*), and density plots (*lower panels*) for two

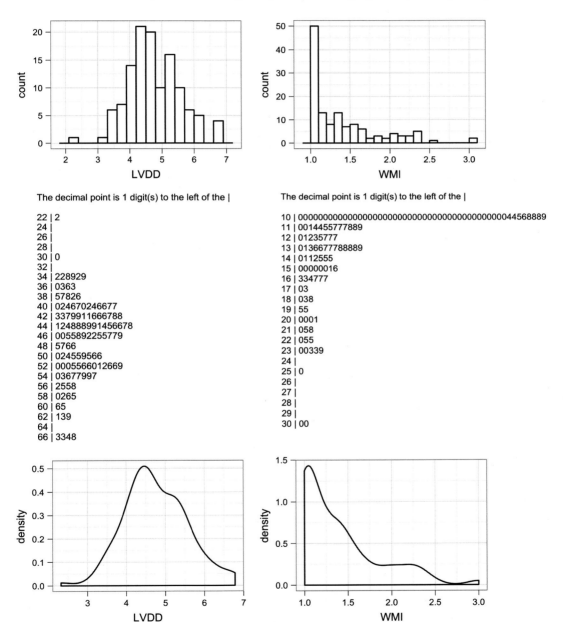

Fig. 3.7 Histograms (*top panels*), stem-and-leaf plots (*central panels*) and density plots (*lower panels*) for the distribution of variables LVDD (left ventricular end-diastolic dimension) and WMI (a measure of how the segments of the left ventricle are moving, divided by the number of segments seen) from the Echocardiogram dataset

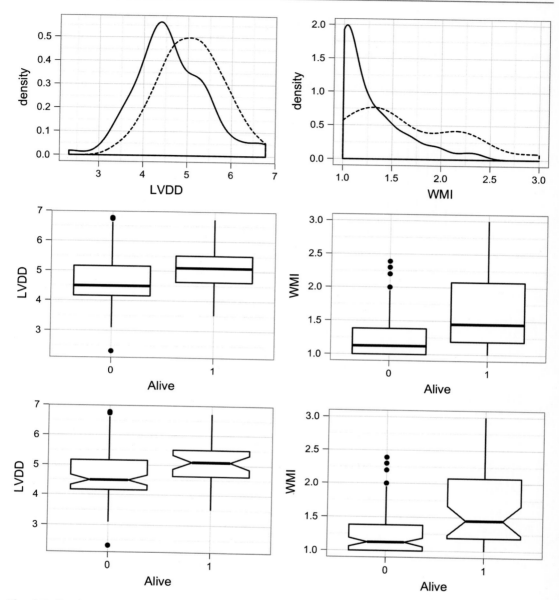

Fig. 3.8 Density plots (*top panels*), boxplots (*center panels*), and notched boxplots for LVDD and WMI for alive (coded with 1) and not-alive patients (coded with 0)

from the Echocardiogram dataset. In density plots (*top panels*), the distributions of the alive patients are reported as *dashed lines*

continuous variables from the Echocardiogram dataset, the left ventricular end-diastolic dimension (LVDD), and a measure of how the segments of the left ventricle are moving divided by the number of segments seen (WMI). All graphical tools show clearly that the two

variables have a very different distribution structure: LVDD appears to be only slightly asymmetric, whereas WMI shows a strong asymmetry with a long right tail. The stem-and-leaf plots and the density plots also suggest that different distributions might have been incorrectly mixed.

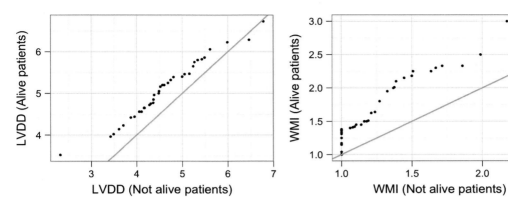

Fig.   3.9 QQplots   for   LVDD   (left   ventricular end-diastolic   dimension;   *left   panel*)   and   WMI (a measure of how the segments of the left ventricle are moving, divided by the number of segments seen; *right panel*) for alive and not-alive patients from the Echocardiogram dataset

Table 3.2   Selected descriptive statistics for LVDD and WMI for alive and not-alive patients from the Echocardiogram dataset

Statistics	LVDD (not alive)	LVDD (alive)	WMI (not alive)	WMI (alive)
Min	2.320	3.520	1.000	1.000
Lower quartile	4.160	4.628	1.000	1.190
Median	4.490	5.105	1.125	1.450
Upper quartile	5.160	5.515	1.382	2.078
Max	6.780	6.730	2.390	3.000
Mean	4.624	5.091	1.258	1.630
MAD	0.726	0.741	0.185	0.638
SD	0.810	0.719	0.335	0.555

To investigate this latter issue, we compare the distributions for the group of alive and not-alive patients at the end of the study period. If the plots are the result of some mixing effect, the distributions of the groups should appear well separated. Indeed, in Fig. 3.8 (*top panels*) the density plots clearly show differences in the two groups. Both the distributions of LVDD and of WMI are shifted to the right. Moreover, the distribution of WMI for alive patients appears to have a completely different shape. In the same figure, we provide parallel boxplots (*central panels*) and notched boxplots (*bottom panels*) obtained by plotting the boxplots on the same scale. The comparison of medians using notched boxplots can be regarded as the graphical analogue of a two-sample *t*-test and one-way ANOVA (if more than two groups are considered), showing a rough difference in the position of the two distributions for alive and not-alive

patients. Again, this appears evident by looking at the QQ plots of the distributions of the variables LVDD and WMI for alive and not-alive patients (Fig. 3.9). Clearly, the distribution for the variable LVDD appears similar in shape but with a different location (points are aligned along a straight line, which is different from the straight line passing through the origin with slope equal to one), whereas the distribution of the variable WMI is completely different for the   two   groups   of   patients,   with   strong differences in location, variability, and shape.

Some selected descriptive statistics for the variables LVDD and WMI for alive and not-alive patients are reported in Table 3.2. The first five lines refer to the five-number summary, whereas the remaining lines refer to the mean, the standard deviation, and the MAD. It is worth noting that the difference in variability for the variable WMI in the two groups when measured

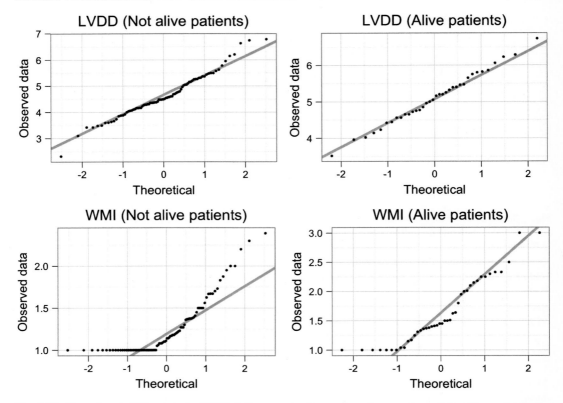

Fig. 3.10 Normal probability plots for LVDD (left ventricular end-diastolic dimension) and WMI (a measure of how the segments of the left ventricle are moving, divided by the number of segments seen) for alive and not-alive patients from the Echocardiogram dataset

by the standard deviation appears much lower than the difference measured by the MAD. This is due to the outlying values, which inflate the measure of spread for the not-alive patients. When no outliers are present, as in the case of LVDD for alive patients, the variability measured by the standard deviation is very close to that measured by the MAD. Please also note that, as this distribution is almost symmetric, the mean and the median are also very close to each other.

The previous discussion strongly supports a general strategy for data analysis that some authors define as "compute and compare": compute more than one statistical tool for each statistical analysis problem and compare the results. This strategy can give invaluable insights into the true structure of the data, since it allows looking at the data from different viewpoints. For instance, both the mean and the median are able to measure the location of a distribution, but they react differently to different characteristics of the dataset. We know they are very close to each other if the distribution is (approximately) symmetric and there are no outliers. So, sensible differences between the two indexes suggest a deeper analysis of the data for possible asymmetry and/or outlying observations. In general, when both robust and non-robust statistical tools are available, a close look at the results gives invaluable hints on the presence of extreme observations. Clearly, this strategy implies a good knowledge of the statistical tools being used with a deep knowledge of the assumptions (implicit or explicit) which, when fulfilled, allow them to deliver accurate and trustable results. This is one reason why blind usage of statistical software can be ineffective or even dangerous.

The normal probability plots for LVDD and WMI for alive and not-alive patients are reported in Fig. 3.10. Clearly, the distribution of the variable WMI is far from normal, whereas—for

Table 3.3 Normality tests (*p*-values in parenthesis) for LVDD and WMI for alive and not-alive patients from the Echocardiogram dataset

Normality tests	LVDD (not alive)	LVDD (alive)	WMI (not alive)	WMI (alive)
Jarque–Bera	3.032 (0.2196)	0.226 (0.8929)	43.517 (0.0000)	4.128 (0.1269)
Shapiro–Wilks	0.977 (0.1338)	0.995 (0.9998)	0.782 (0.0000)	0.902 (0.0016)
Anderson–Darling	0.662 (0.0812)	0.094 (0.9970)	6.542 (0.0000)	1.301 (0.0020)
D'Agostino	3.749 (0.1534)	0.067 (0.9671)	29.101 (0.0000)	4.406 (0.1105)

variable LVDD—the normality assumption appears to be very reasonable (the points are well aligned along the line). This is largely confirmed by the results of the normality tests reported in Table 3.3. All the tests considered support the normality assumption for the LVDD variable (all *p*-values are high and well above the 5 % significance level usually considered). The normality assumption should be rejected, at any level of significance, for the variable WMI for not-alive patients. The results for WMI for the group of alive patients are less clear. In this latter case, the Shapiro–Wilks and the Anderson–Darling tests point toward rejection of the null at the level of significance of 1 %, whereas the JB and the D'Agostino test do not reject the null. This happens because the different tests are constructed to detect specific issues that can imply departure from normality. For instance, the JB test statistic is able to detect departure from normality as long as they impact the skewness and the kurtosis of the data distribution. Other aspects that can affect normality of the variable are not considered at all.

The previous discussion again supports the use of a "compute and compare" strategy. The different tests investigate different aspects of the distribution, can characterize its normality, and may also deliver different results.

Point estimates for the population mean and the population median for the four datasets are reported in Table 3.4. For both LVDD and WMI, there is an increase in sample means and in sample medians when moving from not alive to alive patients. In all cases, the standard error increases as the result of an increase in variability when moving from the not-alive to the alive patients group. Increasing variability appears to be particularly significant for the variable WMI

Table 3.4 Sample mean and sample medians, along with corresponding standard errors, for LVDD and WMI for alive and not-alive patients from the Echocardiogram dataset

Statistics	LVDD		WMI	
	Not alive	Alive	Not alive	Alive
Median	4.49	5.105	1.125	1.45
SE (Median)	0.085	0.12	0.045	0.055
Mean	4.624	5.091	1.258	1.63
SE (Mean)	0.088	0.119	0.036	0.086
n	85	36	88	42

and for the sample mean: in this case, the standard error is more than double for the alive patients with respect to not-alive patients. Figure 3.11 clearly shows the relative merits of the sample mean and the sample medians in estimating the location of a dataset. For symmetric (or nearly symmetric) distributions, the median is very close to the mean, whereas for asymmetric distributions, the median delivers a much better estimate of the "center" of the observed dataset.

Confidence intervals for the population mean and population median are reported in Table 3.5, and their lengths are reported in Table 3.6. As expected, estimates with a greater standard error deliver longer confidence intervals.

To check whether the observed differences in the two samples of alive and not-alive patients are significant or have arisen by chance solely as a consequence of sampling variability, we can test the null hypothesis that the population means in the two groups are equals using a *t*-test (using the Welch version to account for possibly unequal population variances). The results are reported in Table 3.7. The *p*-values of the tests are all very low (well below 1 %), supporting the conclusions that observed differences in the

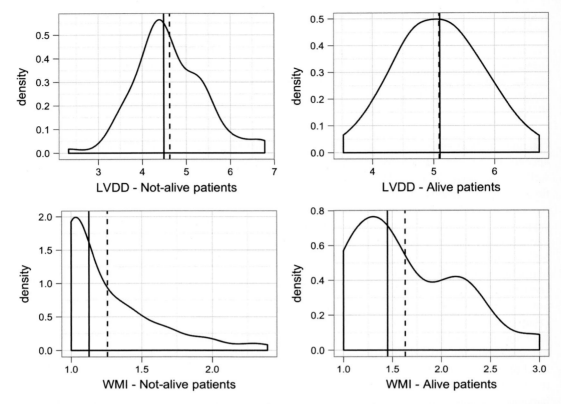

Fig. 3.11 Sample mean and sample medians, along with density estimation, for LVDD (left ventricular end-diastolic dimension) and WMI (a measure of how the segments of the left ventricle are moving, divided by the number of segments seen) for alive and not-alive patients from the Echocardiogram dataset

Table 3.5 95 % confidence intervals for the population means and population medians for LVDD and WMI for alive and not-alive patients from the Echocardiogram dataset

		LVDD		WMI	
Statistics	Method	Not alive	Alive	Not alive	Alive
Median	Asymptotic	(4.301, 4.679)	(4.797, 5.413)	(1.023, 1.227)	(1.320, 1.580)
	Bootstrap	(4.290, 4.620)	(4.820, 5.460)	(1.045, 1.220)	(1.112, 1.535)
Mean	Asymptotic	(4.449, 4.799)	(4.848, 5.335)	(1.187, 1.329)	(1.457, 1.803)
	Bootstrap	(4.448, 4.799)	(4.847, 5.342)	(1.195, 1.340)	(1.468, 1.820)

Asymptotic intervals are based on the standard normal distribution. The basic bootstrap has been used for the median case, whereas the bootstrap-t method has been used for the mean

sample means are not solely due to sampling variability. However, the t-test requires normality assumptions for the two populations, which we already know is reasonable for the variable LVDD but not for the variable WMI. Therefore, we can expect accurate conclusions for the test on LVDD, but we cannot be sure on the results for the test on WMI. Even if we make use of some kind of large sample argument to apply the t-test for non-normal populations, it is a good idea to also compute nonparametric tests (which do not rely on any normality assumption) and compare the results. Quite interestingly, the Mann–Whitney test (the nonparametric counterpart of the t-test) leads to exactly the same conclusions as the t-test. However, different conclusions apply for the two variables. For the variable LVDD, the exploratory analysis

Table 3.6 95 % confidence interval lengths for the population means and population medians for LVDD and WMI for alive and not-alive patients from the Echocardiogram dataset

Statistics	Method	LVDD		WMI	
		Not alive	Alive	Not alive	Alive
Median	Asymptotic	0.378	0.616	0.204	0.260
	Bootstrap	0.330	0.640	0.175	0.423
Mean	Asymptotic	0.350	0.487	0.142	0.352
	Bootstrap	0.351	0.495	0.145	0.344

Table 3.7 Observed values for test statistics and p-values (in parenthesis) of the Welch two-sample t-test and of the Mann–Whitney rank test for LVDD and WMI for alive and not-alive patients from the Echocardiogram dataset

Variable	t-test	Mann–Whitney
LVDD	3.143 (0.0024)	3.133 (0.0015)
WMI	4.011 (0.0002)	4.009 (0.0000)

Table 3.8 Difference in location and 95 % confidence interval for LVDD and WMI for alive and not-alive patients from the Echocardiogram dataset

Variable	Mean difference	Median difference
LVDD	0.467 (0.171, 0.763)	0.490 (0.180, 0.797)
WMI	0.372 (0.186, 0.558)	0.320 (0.150, 0.455)

suggests that the distributions in the two groups are comparable in shape: they have similar variability and the same parent distribution (Gaussian). The only difference appears to be in location. So the Mann–Whitney test is actually supporting a shift in the location (measured by the median) of the distribution of alive patients with respect to not-alive patients. Conversely, the distribution of the variable WMI in the two groups is significantly different. Consequently, the results of the Mann–Whitney test also reflect this circumstance.

Estimates of the difference in location for the variables LVDD and WMI (along with the corresponding 95 % confidence intervals) are reported in Table 3.8.

Lessons Learned

Statistical analysis involves "learning from experience" and plays a central role in applied research, including biomedical research. The three basic statistical concepts—data collection, summary, and inference—are deeply embedded in any research workflow.

Study design and data collection are key issues for successful statistical analysis, and the key point is how to tailor the study design to the research objectives. In most cases, researchers work on samples, but they wish to extrapolate the results from a study to the population in general. In this respect, two issues are particularly important: for observational studies, the observed samples should be selected in such a way that guarantees they are representative of the populations of interest; for experimental or case–control studies, groups being compared should be as similar as possible apart from the features of direct interest.

Data from a well-planned design can be analyzed in several alternative ways with a great number of statistical tools, leading researchers to meaningful conclusions. However, no sophisticated statistical analysis is able to compensate for problems with poor study designs.

The easy access to user-friendly and powerful statistical software may tempt researchers to attempt complex statistical modeling. However, this approach may imply the use of inappropriate statistical tools, which in turn may lead to erroneous conclusions. Conversely, simple descriptive statistical measures and well-chosen plots can provide invaluable insight into the structure of the sample. This deeper understanding of the data allows practitioners to both choose appropriate statistical tools and draw meaningful conclusions from the observed data.

In addition, any statistical analysis should include accurate data checking to ensure all data recorded are plausible. This should be easy for categorical data, since there are (usually) a small number of prespecified values; for continuous data, usually only range checking is possible. After data are checked and all gross errors are amended, it is important to screen the data to identify features that may cause difficulties during the statistical analysis. Basically, data should be checked for missing data and outlying observations and whether data transformation is necessary to meet the required assumptions.

Both numerical summaries and appropriate graphical tools should be used in this exploratory step, as it is well known that "a graph is worth a thousand words." Moreover, since outlying observations might be present in the dataset, both conventional and robust techniques should be employed. By comparing the results of different statistical tools known to be valid under different assumptions, the researcher can obtain invaluable insights into the true structure of the data. This "compute and compare" strategy should become the standard practice of any data analyst.

Confidence intervals are a fundamental tool for inference, as they can deliver information about the estimate of a population characteristic, along with its accuracy. The use of confidence intervals in reporting the results of biomedical research has increased dramatically over the past several years. The standard approach for computing a confidence interval for the population mean is based on the Student's t-distribution or on the Gaussian approximation. For data sampled from a symmetric and light-tailed distribution (i.e., a distribution close to the Gaussian), the empirical coverage probability (i.e., the proportion of the confidence intervals that contains the population parameter being estimated over many studies) is close to the nominal confidence level. However, for symmetric but heavy-tailed distributions, the empirical coverage tends to be higher than the nominal level. Even worse, for skewed distributions, empirical coverage can be poor and large samples might be necessary to obtain reasonable results. Bootstrap methods can be a valid and effective alternative to asymptotic approximations based on Gaussian distributions. They can provide more accurate confidence intervals, especially for small and moderate sample sizes, under quite general conditions, which are fulfilled in most practical cases.

Moving to statistical tests to compare two populations, the analyst should be aware that selecting the right statistical test may be difficult, but a good knowledge and understanding of the characteristics of the dataset and of the population under study may lead to the correct decision. It is important to know at least whether (1) the datasets are random samples; (2) the data are paired or independent; (3) the populations are Gaussian. In particular, if the data are drawn from Gaussian populations, the classical t-test will deliver accurate results. This remains true for large samples; however, for non-Gaussian populations and for small and moderate sample sizes, it is advisable to employ nonparametric methods, which are known to be valid under much weaker and more general conditions.

For confidence intervals and hypothesis testing, again, a "compute and compare" strategy is suggested. Significant differences between the results of classic parametric approaches and nonparametric approaches may suggest interesting data characteristics of which the analyst was not aware.

Statistical analysis cannot be conducted without using some sort of statistical software. However, the choice of software must be carefully planned, taking into account the budget (including license, maintenance, and training costs), the specific statistical needs (general purpose and/or specific software), the future scaling needs (both in terms of amount of data and of statistical techniques needed), and the workflow of the research unit.

References

1. Altman DG. Practical statistics for medical research. London: Chapman and Hall; 1991.
2. Kirkwood BR, Sterne JA. Essential medical statistics. 2nd ed. Hoboken: Blackwell Science; 2003.

3. Wayne WD. Biostatistics. A foundation for analysis in the health science. Hoboken, NJ: Wiley; 2005.
4. Wilcox RR. Introduction to robust estimation and hypothesis testing. 2nd ed. San Diego, CA: Academic; 2005.
5. Wilcox RR. Fundamentals of modern statistical methods. 2nd ed. New York: Springer; 2010.
6. Wilcox RR. Basic Statistics. Understanding conventional methods and modern insights. Oxford: Oxford University Press; 2010.
7. Machin D, Campbell MJ. Design of studies for medical research. Chichester: John Wiley and Sons Ltd.; 2005.
8. Tillé Y. Sampling algorithms. New York: Springer; 2006.
9. Rosenberger JL, Gasko M. Comparing location estimators: trimmed means, medians and trimean. In: Hoaglin DC, Mosteller F, Tukey JW, editors. Understanding Robust and Exploratory Data Analysis. New York: Wiley; 1983. p. 293–338.
10. Croux C, Rousseeuw PJ. Time-efficient algorithms for two highly robust estimators of scale. In: Doge Y, Whittaker J, editors. Computational statistics, vol. 1. Heidelberg: Physica-Verlag; 1992. p. 411–28.
11. Rousseeuw PJ, Croux C. Alternatives to median absolute deviation. J Am Stat Assoc. 1993;88 (424):1273–83.
12. Horn PS, Feng L, Li Y, Pesce AJ. Effect of outliers and nonhealthy individuals on reference interval estimation. Clin Chem. 2001;47(12):2137–45.
13. Barnett V, Lewis T. Outliers in statistical data. 3rd ed. New York: John Wiley and Sons Ltd.; 1994.
14. Atkinson AC, Riani M, Cerioli A. Exploring multivariate data with the forward search. New York: Springer; 2004.
15. Hadi AS, Imon AHMR, Werner M. Detection of outliers. WIREs Comp Stat. 2009;1:57–70. doi:10.1002/wics.6.
16. Solberg HE, Lahti A. Detection of outliers in reference distributions: Performance of horn's algorithm. Clin Chem. 2005;51(12):2326–32.
17. Hodge VJ, Austin J. A survey of outlier detection methodologies. Artif Intell Rev. 2004;22(2):85–126.
18. Fritsch V, Varoquaux G, Thyreau B, Poline JB, Thirion B. Detecting outliers in high-dimensional neuroimaging datasets with robust covariance estimators. Medical image analysis. Forthcoming 2012. doi: 10.1016/j.media.2012.05.002.
19. Maronna RA, Martin DR, Yohai VJ. Robust statistics. Theory and methods. Chichester: John Wiley and Sons Ltd.; 2006.
20. Woolrich M. Robust group analysis using outlier inference. Neuroimage. 2008;41:286–301.
21. Chambers JM, Cleveland WS, Kleiner B, Tukey PA. Graphical methods for data analysis. Belmont, CA: Wadsworth; 1983.
22. Bowman AW, Azzalini A. Applied smoothing techniques for data analysis. Oxford: Clarendon; 1997.
23. McGill R, Tukey JW, Larsen WA. Variations of box plots. Am Stat. 1978;32(1):12–6.
24. Tukey JW. Exploratory data analysis. London: Pearson; 1977.
25. Yazici B, Yolacan S. A comparison of various tests of normality. J Stat Comput Simul. 2007;77 (2):175–83.
26. Thode HC. Testing for normality. New York: Marcel Dekker; 2002.
27. Osborne JW. Improving your data transformations: applying the Box-Cox transformation. Pract Assess Res Eval. 2010;15(12):1–9.
28. Lehmann EL. Nonparametrics. Statistical methods based on ranks. New York: Springer; 2006.
29. Olive DJ. A Simple Confidence Interval for the Median. Preprint available from www.math.siu.edu/olive/ppmedci.pdf. 2005.
30. Efron B. Bootstrap methods: another look at the jackknife. Ann Stat. 1979;7:1–26.
31. Efron B, Tibshirani RJ. An introduction to the bootstrap. London: Chapman and Hall; 1993.
32. Hall P. On the number of bootstrap simulations required to construct a confidence interval. Ann Stat. 1986;14:1453–62.
33. Carpenter J, Bithell J. Bootstrap confidence intervals: when, which, what? A practical guide for medical statisticians. Stat Med. 2000;19:1141–64.
34. Davidson AC, Hinkley DV. Bootstrap Methods and their Application. Cambridge: Cambridge University Press; 1997.
35. Armitage P, Berry G. Statistical methods in medical research. Oxford: Blackwell Science; 2002.
36. Hollander M, Wolfe DA. Nonparametric statistical methods. 2nd ed. New York: John Wiley & Sons; 1999.
37. Hart A. (2001) Mann-Whitney test is not just a test of medians: differences in spread can be important. BMJ. 2001;323:391–3.
38. Shao J, Tu D. The jackknife and bootstrap. New York: Springer; 1995.
39. Bauer DF. Constructing confidence sets using rank statistics. J Am Stat Assoc. 1972;67:687–90.
40. Rodriguez RN. SAS. WIREs Comp Stat. 2011;3:1–11. doi:10.1002/wics.131.
41. Hilbe JM. A review of Stata 9.0. Am Stat. 2005;59 (4):335–48.
42. Gutierrez RG. STATA. WIREs Comp Stat. 2010;2:728–33. doi:10.1002/wics.116.
43. Hilbe JM. Systat 12.2. Am Stat. 2008;62(2):177–8.
44. Hilbe JM. A review of Systat 11. Am Stat. 2005;59 (1):104–10.
45. Hilbe JM. STATISTICA 7. Am Stat. 2007;61 (1):91–4.
46. Jones B, Sall J. JMP statistical discovery software. WIREs Comp Stat. 2011;3:188–94. doi:10.1002/wics.162.
47. Wilkinson L. SYSTAT. WIREs Comp Stat. 2010;2:256–7. doi:10.1002/wics.66.

48. McCullogh BD, Wilson B. On the accuracy of statistical procedures in Microsoft Excel 2000 and Excel XP. Comput Stat Data Anal. 2002;40:713–21.

49. R Core Team. R: A language and environment for statistical computing. R Foundation for Statistical Computing, Vienna, Austria. 2012. ISBN 3-900051-07-0, URL http://www.R-project.org/

50. McCullogh BD, Wilson B. On the accuracy of statistical procedures in Microsoft Excel 2003. Comput Stat Data Anal. 2005;49:1244–52.

51. McCullogh BD, Heiser DA. On the accuracy of statistical procedures in Microsoft Excel 2007. Comput Stat Data Anal. 2008;52:4570–8.

52. Frank A, Asuncion A. UCI machine learning repository [http://archive.ics.uci.edu/ml]. Irvine, CA: University of California, School of Information and Computer Science; 2010.

Part II
Applications

Microscopy Techniques

4

Antonia Feola, Letizia Cito, Angelina Di Carlo,
Alfonso Giovane, and Marina Di Domenico

Phase Contrast

Phase contrast microscopy is a contrast-enhancing optical technique that can be applied to unstained biological specimens because it improves the contrast images of transparent specimens without affecting resolution. It is mainly used to examine dynamic events in living cells [1–7].

Two parameters should be considered in phase contrast microscopy: the light wave amplitude and the light wave phase. Changes in amplitude are due to the absorption or scattering of light. The human eye is only sensitive to amplitude variations that are perceived as changes in brightness and cannot perceive changes in phase. The technique is based on an optical mechanism that converts light phase variations to changes in amplitude, which can be visualized as differences in image contrast. To make phase changes visible in phase contrast microscopy, the illuminating light background is separated from the specimen's scattered light. In a normal microscope, the illumination of an unstained biological specimen produces a weak scattered light, the phase of which is usually shifted by 90°, resulting in a low-contrast image. In the phase contrast microscope, the phase of background light is shifted by 90° by passing it through a phase shift ring. Thus, the phase difference between the background and the scattered light is eliminated, producing an increased contrast. One of the advantages of phase contrast microscopy is that living cells can be examined in their natural state without killing, fixing, and staining them [8–10]. This technique enables the observation and recording of biological processes in high contrast with sharp clarity [11–14]. Prior to the invention of phase contrast techniques, transmitted bright field illumination was one of the most commonly used tools in optical microscopy, especially for fixed stained specimens or other types of samples showing high natural absorption of visible light. The addition of phase contrast optical accessories to a standard bright field microscope can be

A. Feola (✉)
Department of Biology, University of Naples "Federico II", Via Cinthia, 2, 80126 Naples, Italy
e-mail: antonia.feola@unina.it

L. Cito
INT-CROM, "Pascale Foundation" National Cancer Institute-Cancer Research Center, 83013 Mercogliano, Italy
e-mail: letizia.cito@cro-m.eu

A. Di Carlo
Department of Medico Surgical Sciences and Biotechnologies, University of Rome "Sapienza", Corso della Repubblica, 79, 04100 Latina, Italy
e-mail: angelina.dicarlo@uniroma.it

A. Giovane • M. Di Domenico
Department of Biochemistry, Biophysics and General Pathology, Seconda Università degli Studi di Napoli, Via de Crecchio, 7, 80138 Naples, Italy
e-mail: alfonso.giovane@unina2.it;
marina.didomenico@unina2.it

© Springer Science+Business Media New York 2016
F.M. Sacerdoti et al. (eds.), *Advanced Imaging Techniques in Clinical Pathology*,
Current Clinical Pathology, DOI 10.1007/978-1-4939-3469-0_4

49

employed as a technique to render a contrast-enhancing effect in transparent specimens, similar to optical staining. So far, modern phase contrast microscopes enable the detection of specimens with very small internal structures, or even just a few protein molecules, when the technology is coupled to electronic enhancement and post-acquisition image processing [15–17].

Differential Interference Contrast (DIC)

Differential interference contrast (DIC) is a mechanism for enhancing contrast in transparent specimens. It produces contrast by visually showing the refractive index gradients of different areas of a specimen. The invention in 1950 is attributed to Georges Nomarski, who modified the Wollaston prism. The modification consists in cutting one edge of the prism in such a manner that the optical axis is oriented obliquely with respect to the flat surface of the prism. This modification causes the light rays to come to a focal point outside the body of the prism. The light beam is polarized and then split into two separate beams, the distance of which is equal to the resolution of the objective lens. One beam path is directed through the specimen and the other acts as a reference beam; the two beams are then combined. Since different parts of the specimen have different refractive indices, when the beams are gathered by a second polarizing filter, the vibrational planes of the beams is restored; this causes variations in amplitude that are visualized as differences in brightness [18–25].

DIC microscopy has the following advantages:

- It is possible to make fuller use of the numerical aperture of the system.
- There are no confusing halos.
- Images can be seen in striking color (optical staining) and with a 3D shadow-like appearance. The visibility of outlines and details is greatly improved, and the photomicrography of these images is striking in color and detail.

- Regular planachromats or achromats (also suitable for ordinary bright-field work) can be used if the manufacturer states that such objectives are designed for their apparatus.

DIC also has the following disadvantages or limitations:

- The equipment for DIC is quite expensive because of the many prisms that are required.
- Birefringent specimens, such as those found in many kinds of crystals, may not be suitable because of their effect on polarized light. Similarly, specimen carriers, such as culture vessels and Petri dishes made of plastic may not be suitable. For such specimens, Hoffman modulation contrast may be a better choice.
- Apochromatic objectives may not be suitable because such objectives themselves may significantly affect polarized light.
- For very thin or scattered specimens, better images may be achieved using phase contrast methods. DIC microscopy has been used to assess the new bone formation and microstructure [26], to detect retinitis pigmentosa [27], to measure the lamellarity of giant lipid vesicles [28], to quantify volume, mass, and density of thrombus formation [29]. Furthermore, three-dimensional imaging of cell division and analysis of microtubule dynamic were studied by this technique [30, 31].

Wide-Field Fluorescence

Wide-field fluorescence or epi-fluorescence microscopy is a common technique used to acquire both topographical and dynamic information. It is based on the irradiation of the whole sample with a light of a specific wavelength, and the weaker emitted fluorescence is then separated from the stronger excitation light. The microscope is configured in such a way that only the emission light can reach the detector or eye. The resulting fluorescent image is superimposed with high contrast against a black

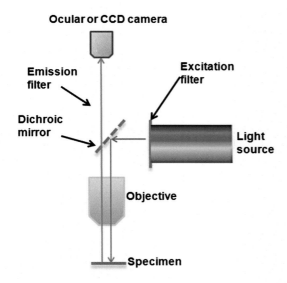

Fig. 4.1 Schematic representation of a wide-field microscope

background. The limits of detection are generally regulated by the contrast between the fluorescent image and the darkness of the background. A fluorescence microscope, as shown in Fig. 4.1, basically constitutes an arc lamp (usually a mercury or xenon), an optical tube containing exciting filters producing a defined band of wavelengths, a dichroic mirror (which has the ability to reflect excitation wavelengths and pass emission wavelengths), and an emission filter (also known as a barrier filter). These three components are the heart of the system and are usually assembled by the manufacturer in a block or cube to give the right monochromatic light beam to produce the best signal-to-noise ratio. The light emerging from the emission filter is then captured by an observation tube that can be connected to an eyepiece or a digital camera. The excitation light is directed onto the specimen by passing it through the selected excitation filter and then through the microscope objective, which acts as a condenser. The light beam reaches the specimen, the emitted fluorescence then passes through the same objective, reaching the ocular or the digital camera. Therefore, both the illumination and the detection of light take place simultaneously and cover the whole visual field, depending on the microscope objective.

Filters play a fundamental role in fluorescence microscopy, with two types generally used: a band-pass filter and a long pass filter. The band-pass filter transmits a light of a discrete wavelength that has a maximum centered in the range of 20–40 nm. The long pass filter cuts off the light lower than a certain wavelength and transmits light higher than that wavelength.

The excitation filter is usually a band-pass filter that passes only light of the right wavelength for fluorophore excitation. The emission or barrier filter is generally a long pass filter and separates fluorescence produced by the fluorophore from background light. The barrier filter transmits light of the fluorescence wavelength coming from the dichroic mirror while blocking all other light from the excitation lamp (reflected from the specimen or optical elements). This is necessary because the intensity of fluorescent light is about 100,000-fold weaker than the excitation light.

The dichroic mirror is a filter and a mirror at the same time because it reflects the light coming from the excitation filter and passes the fluorescent light coming from the specimen. A dichroic mirror used in an epi-fluorescence microscope is placed at 45° with respect to the excitation light, which is reflected 90° toward the objective and the specimen. The fluorescence light coming from the specimen passes through the dichroic mirror, directed toward the observer (or high-sensitivity camera) [32–34].

Fluorescence is usually used to increase the sensitivity of different techniques. When a light beam of a certain energy $E_i = h\nu_i$ interacts with a fluorescent molecule, it can be absorbed if its energy is equal to or greater than the energy necessary to promote a quantum leap of an electron belonging to that molecule. The electron in the excited state decays to the ground state by emitting a radiative energy $E_{em} = h\nu_{em}$ were h is the Planck constant and ν is the frequency. Since most fluorophores have a larger dipole moment in the excited state than in the ground state, the solvent molecules can reorient around the excited molecule, lowering its energy. Thus, E_{em} becomes lesser than E_i and $\nu_{em} < \nu_i$ but frequency is inversely proportional to wavelength according to the equation $c = \nu\lambda$ (where

c is the light velocity). Thus, the emission light has a longer wavelength of exciting light; this phenomenon is known as Stokes shift. The dimension of the shift depends on the molecular structure, which ranges from a few nanometers to several hundred nanometers. Generally, fluorophores used in microscopy range between 20 and 100 nm. The occurrence of Stokes shift is critical to an increase in sensitivity of fluorescence imaging measurements. The emission shift allows the use of optical filters with a bandwidth that efficiently blocks excitation light from reaching the detector; therefore, the relatively low fluorescence signal can be observed with a low-noise background.

In addition to the Stokes shift, other parameters are important in defining fluorophores, as follows:

The extinction coefficient (ε)
The fluorescence lifetime (τ)
The quantum yield (Φ)

The molar extinction coefficient ε is defined as the absorption produced by a 1 M solution of a substance at a particular wavelength (usually that of maximum absorption), determined in a cuvette of 1 cm path length. Extinction coefficient is a direct measure of the ability of a molecule to absorb light; fluorophores with a high extinction coefficient also have a high probability of high fluorescence emission.

The fluorescence lifetime τ is the time that a molecule remains in an excited state prior to returning to the ground state. Because the lifetime of a fluorophore is inversely proportional to the extinction coefficient, molecules with a high extinction coefficient have an excited state with a short lifetime. Fluorescence intensity is proportional to the number of molecules in the excited state; however, in the excited state, a molecule possesses a dipolar moment that can be perturbed by several factors such as solvent polarity, collision with other molecules in the ground state, temperature, and pH. These factors contribute to the relaxation of the excited state dispersing its energy in a non-radiative form, thus decreasing fluorescence intensity (this decrease is called fluorescence quenching). The parameter that describes the fluorescence intensity is the quantum yield Φ, which is the ratio between the photons emitted and the photons absorbed. As calculated, this parameter has a dimensionless value ranging between 0 and 1; however, the value almost never reaches 1. Quantum yield is the fluorescence equivalent of the molar extinction; fluorophores with high quantum yield produce a more intense signal, thus increasing the measure sensitivity. However, care should be taken in measuring the fluorescence intensity of probes in living cells because it may change according to the cellular district because of differing pH or polarity. Photobleaching is another event that affects fluorescence. This phenomenon, while not yet completely understood, is responsible for a decrease in fluorescence from a long irradiation of molecules and seems to be due to the interaction of oxygen with the excited fluorophore. In fact, the oxygen dissolved in the sample medium can interact in its triplet ground state with a particular excited state of the fluorophore in which a cross from singlet to triplet status occurs. Since the molecule in the triplet state has a lifetime of a millisecond—versus the nanosecond in singlet state—it can interact with oxygen for longer, generating an oxygen radical. The oxygen radical reacts with the more reactive fluorophore in its excited state, thus quenching the fluorescence [35].

Fluorescence microscopy is now one of the most used techniques in biology, thanks to the availability of a large number of fluorophores (also named dyes) synthesized to respond to several characteristics such as high quantum yield, large Stokes shift, and resistance to photobleaching.

Dyes can be modified to bind to specific biological targets. A dye modified in this manner is called a probe. Several probes are synthesized to monitor the most diverse biological functions in living cells, such as chelation to ions, pH sensitivity, and lipid transport and metabolism [36–42]. Furthermore, a dye can be linked to an antibody to study a localization of a specific protein in a fixed cell or tissue [43]. Moreover, fluorescence microscopy can also be used for DNA imaging [44, 45]. However, if different probes are used simultaneously, several target molecules can be identified in the same specimen.

Confocal Microscopy

Confocal microscopy has significant advantages over wide-field microscopy. In particular, it can produce images with reduced degradation as most of the out-of-focus light from the specimen is removed [46]. Furthermore, this technique enables the acquisition of a series of optical sections along the thickness of the specimen (z axis). In a wide-field fluorescence microscope, the fluorescence emitted by the specimen comes from that emitted not only by the focal plane but also by the layers up and down it, producing an out-of-focus fluorescent light that decreases the image resolution.

Basically, wide-field and confocal microscopes have the same optical light path; however, several differences are encountered along this light path. First, the light beam is generated by a laser source that produces a coherent beam with a greater intensity and a reduced bandwidth. The term "laser" is an acronym of "*l*ight *a*mplification by *s*timulated *e*mission of *r*adiation." Laser light is different from other light sources by virtue of its coherence, which allows the laser beam to be focused to a tight spot, and the narrow beam has limited diffraction. The light beam, like the wide-field microscope, is reflected by a dichroic mirror and passes through the objective, to focus on a very small region of the specimen. The fluorescence emitted by the irradiated point on the specimen passes through the dichroic mirror and reaches the pinhole located just before the emission filter and the detector. This alignment allows the pinhole and the irradiated surface of the specimen to be on the same focal plane (confocal). Thus, only the fluorescence emitted from the specimen surface in the confocal plane can pass through the pinhole, whereas fluorescent light from the specimen regions other than the focal plane is excluded. Moreover, in wide-field fluorescence microscopy, the whole specimen is subject to irradiation of an incoherent light, and the image produced by fluorescence emission can be directly observed in the eyepiece or acquired by a charge-coupled device (CCD) camera. In a confocal fluorescence microscope, the image is produced by scanning the specimen surface with a laser beam and simultaneously acquiring the fluorescent light emission through a photomultiplier so the fluorescence intensity coming from each point scanned is registered by a computer and the whole image is reconstituted via dedicated software. For this purpose, the confocal microscope is equipped with a scan head with optical and electronic components. In fact, the scan head moves the laser beam along the xy axes of the specimen, collects the corresponding fluorescence emission, and sends it to the photomultiplier. When a new specimen region along the z axis is focused, the new region becomes confocal to the observed region on the detector. Thus, images of different specimen slices along the z axis can be obtained and a 3D image can be reconstituted using appropriate software [47, 48].

With respect to the wide-field microscope, excitation and fluorescence intensity can be regulated in several ways in the confocal microscope. In fact, varying the laser energy can regulate the exciting light intensity; fluorescence intensity can be controlled by changing the pinhole diameter and by the photomultiplier gain. Generally, a measurement is a compromise between resolution and sensitivity; this is also true for confocal microscopy. In fact, to increase resolution, the pinhole diameter must be very narrow. Whereas, on one hand, a narrow aperture allows fewer out-of-focus photons to reach the photomultiplier, it also reduces the number of confocal photons reaching the detector, decreasing fluorescence intensity and therefore sensitivity. However, fluorescence intensity can be increased in two ways: by increasing the laser energy or the photomultiplier gain. In the first case, increasing the laser energy produces two negative effects: it increases autofluorescence and photobleaching. In the second case, the increase in gain also increases the background currents of the photomultiplier, thus reducing the signal-to-noise ratio, which affects resolution. Therefore, if only a qualitative determination is required, all these effects hardly affect the measure. However, if a quantitative measurement is

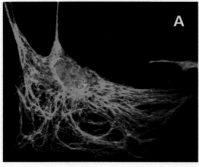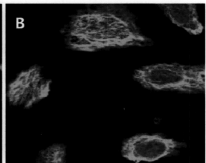

Fig. 4.2 Dual (**a**) and triple (**b**) staining confocal imaging of endothelial cells. (**a**) Vimentin (*green*) and the nuclear protein P16 (*red*) were stained. (**b**) Same as (**a**) but nuclei are stained with DAPI (*blue*). Cell images were acquired via oil-immersed objective (63×), but image (**a**) was further magnified via digital zoom

needed, care should be taken when measuring the fluorescence intensity of the control and the sample with the same microscope settings [49]. Figure 4.2 shows two images of endothelial cells acquired by a confocal microscope stained with double or triple color.

Balestrieri et al. [50] investigated the expression of platelet-activating factor (PAF) receptors in endothelial progenitor cells (EPCs). They demonstrated the presence of PAF receptors by monitoring a transient increase of cytoplasmic Ca^{2+} upon PAF stimulation. The Ca^{2+} transient increase was assessed via laser scanning confocal microscopy in a time-lapse acquisition mode using Fluo 4-AM, a probe that increases its fluorescence when chelated by calcium ions (Fig. 4.3). Confocal microscopy was found useful in elucidating cell organization [51, 52] as well as the molecular mechanisms of neoplastic processes [53–60].

Fig. 4.3 Increase of intracellular Ca^{2+} levels induced by platelet-activating factor (PAF) in the presence and absence of CV3988, a PAF antagonist. Confocal imaging of cells loaded with fluorescent Fluo 4-AM was undertaken using a Zeiss LSM510 system equipped with a 20× (NA) objective. Ca^{2+} ion was measured in time drive configuration (488 nm excitation, 530 nm emission LP510 nm) for 50 slices (about 600 s). In each slice, the fluorescence intensity average was measured by ImageJ free software (http://imagej.nih.gov/ij/)

Total Internal Reflection Fluorescence Microscopy (TIRFM)

Total internal reflection fluorescence microscopy (TIRFM) is based on an optical effect produced by passing a light beam at a high incident angle through glass (i.e., a coverslip) or plastic (i.e., a Petri dish) [61]. The difference in refractive indexes between the glass and the water determines the amount of refraction or reflection light at the interface as a function of beam incident angle. At a specific angle of the glass (or plastic)–water interface, the light beam is totally reflected according to a phenomenon described by Snell that can be summarized by the following equation:

$$n_1 \sin \theta_1 = n_2 \sin \theta_2$$

where n_1 is the medium with the higher refractive index (1.518 for glass microscope slide or coverslip) and n_2 is the medium of the lower refractive index (1.33–1.37 for aqueous buffers). When a light beam impacts upon a medium with an angle θ_1 with respect to the normal, it is refracted with

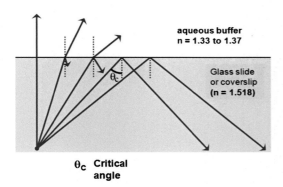

aqueous buffer
n = 1.33 to 1.37

Glass slide
or coverslip
(n = 1.518)

θ_c

θ_C **Critical
angle**

Fig. 4.4 Schematic representation of a light beam reaching the critical angle

an angle θ_2 at the interface into the medium of the lesser refractive index. As the angle θ_1 increases, the beam reaches the critical angle where the refraction is 90°; when the light beam exceeds the critical angle, it is completely reflected at the interface, giving the total internal reflection (Fig. 4.4).

The light reflected generates an electromagnetic field with the same frequency as the incident light; this is called the evanescent wave [62, 63]. Since this wave is produced by a very small (about 200 nm) electromagnetic field and its intensity decreases exponentially with distance, only fluorophores located near the glass–liquid interface can be excited [64, 65]. Thus, fluorophores not in the primary focal plane are not excited; consequently, unwanted secondary fluorescence emission is markedly reduced. This effect produces high-contrast images of the specimen surface with a considerable increase in signal-to-background ratio compared with classical wide-field microscopy [66]. Figure 4.5 is a schematic picture of a TIRF microscope.

In theory, the excitation light could be produced by an arc lamp, but directing the light beam to an appropriate angle while maintaining a suitable intensity is difficult, so a coherent light produced by a laser source is more useful. To obtain a high angle of incidence, the laser irradiates the specimen through the objective lens from the periphery of the back focal plane. The light passes through the objective immersion oil and glass, which have higher refractive indexes than the aqueous media in which cells are immersed. The light is totally reflected according to Snell's law, but a small amount of energy passes through the interface into the lower refractive index media in the form of an evanescent wave that penetrates the specimen, typically 50–100 nm. Only the fluorescent molecules reached by the evanescent wave will be visible, enabling very selective, high-contrast fluorescence imaging. Recently, TIRFM has been used for single-molecule imaging because the background noise, which is a major problem during single-molecule imaging in an aqueous environment, can be overcome by limiting the illumination of excitation light to very near the glass surface. In this way, noise derived from Raman scattering of water molecules and out-of-focus fluorophores is dramatically reduced. The single-molecule imaging technique has already been applied successfully to a wide range of biological systems [67]. It is especially useful in studying the interaction between a ligand and a receptor on the cell surface, cell adhesion onto a surface [68], membrane dynamic or cellular secretion, electron transport in the mitochondrial membrane, cytoskeletal and membrane dynamics [69–73], cellular secretion events [74, 75], and ion transports [76, 77]. TIRF is also useful in studying the conformational dynamics of proteins or binding and triggering of cells by hormones.

Förster Resonance Energy Transfer (FRET)

Förster resonance energy transfer (FRET) is used to study inter- and intra-molecular interactions in living cells and is based on the transfer of non-radiative energy from a donor to an accepting fluorophore.

The resonance energy transfer process can occur when a fluorophore in its excited state, acting as a donor, transfers its excitation energy to an acceptor fluorophore. The transfer is due to a long-range dipole–dipole intermolecular coupling and is satisfied if the fluorescence emission spectrum of the donor overlaps that of the acceptor fluorophore, and the two probes are within a

Fig. 4.5 Schematic picture of a total internal reflection fluorescence microscope

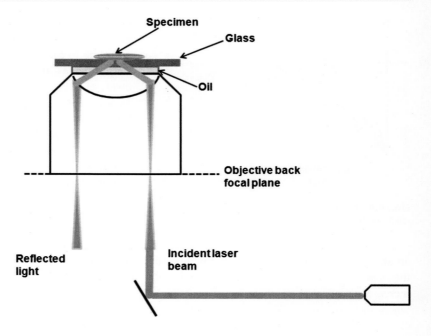

minimal spatial radius of 10 nm. In fact, according to the Förster equation, the transfer depends on the molecular distance at an inverse sixth power:

$$K_{\mathrm{T}} = (1/t_{\mathrm{D}}) \cdot [R_0/r]^6$$

where R_0 is the Förster critical distance, t_{D} is the donor lifetime in the absence of the acceptor, and r is the distance separating the donor and acceptor chromophores.

The Förster critical distance R_0 is defined as the acceptor–donor separation distance for which the transfer rate is equal to the rate of donor decay in the absence of an acceptor. This means that, at a Förster critical distance, 50 % of the donor excitation energy is transferred to the acceptor, whereas the remaining energy is dissipated through fluorescence emission or a thermal process [78, 79].

Besides studies of intermolecular and intramolecular mechanisms, FRET has also been used to explore structural and functional modifications in lipids and proteins. However, this technique requires the use of appropriate fluorophores to label specific targets in living cells; this problem has been overcome in some cases by cloning the jellyfish green fluorescent protein (GFP). GFP can be converted via site-directed mutagenesis into a blue fluorescent protein (BFP) [80]. GFP and BFP mutants possess the fluorescence characteristics to be employed in FRET experiments. Furthermore, FRET microscopy has been extended to the imaging of multiple donor–acceptor pairs by means of a three-fluorophore system using blue, yellow, and red fluorescent proteins [81]. Coupled with advances in pulsed lasers, microscope optics, and computer-based imaging technology, the development of labeling techniques in which the donor and acceptor fluorophores are actually part of the biomolecules themselves has enabled the visualization of dynamic protein interactions within living cells. In addition to the investigation of protein partner interactions, FRET has recently also been applied in studies of protease activity, alterations in membrane voltage potential, calcium metabolism, and the conduction of high-throughput screening assays, such as for quantification of gene expression in single living cells. FRET can also be used to study nucleic acid structural dynamics and the conformational diversity of nucleic acid structure hybridization

[82–84]. FRET is also used in a melting assay that allows the testing of libraries of compounds against different nucleic acid structures to determine whether they stabilize preformed structures [82].

Various examples of FRET use may be found in the scientific literature. Between 1997 and 1998, FRET was used to study Bax and BCL-2 interaction as well as their role in tumorigenesis and apoptosis.

More recently, FRET has been used to analyze the growth processes of axons, and thus the effects of sphingolipids on cerebrovascular permeability and the activation of macrophages by airway mucus. Therefore, FRET is still an effective way to investigate molecular interactions [81, 85–96]. Figure 1 provides an example of images and data gained by FRET.

Fluorescence Recovery After Photobleaching (FRAP)

Photobleaching is a photodynamic event and generally an unwanted phenomenon in fluorescence microscopy because it reduces the intensity of the probe fluorescence. Photobleaching involves the interaction of the fluorophore with a combination of light and oxygen after lengthy irradiation of molecules. The oxygen radical reacts with the more reactive excited fluorophore. The amount of photobleaching is a function of the molecular oxygen concentration and the distance between the fluorophore, oxygen molecules, and other cellular components. Reactions between fluorophores and molecular oxygen permanently destroy fluorescence, quenching light emission.

However, this quenching can be used in FRAP investigations to determine the kinetics of diffusion in living cells [97–103]. In fact, if a small portion of the cell is subjected to lengthy irradiation, the fluorescence in that area is completely quenched. The diffusion or active movement of molecules within the cell then replace the bleached fluorophore with unbleached molecules that were located in a different part of the cell and thus restore the fluorescence. By monitoring the intensity of the fluorescence emission, the translational mobility of a probe can be determined within a very small (2–5 μm) region of a single cell or section of living tissue.

Requirements for FRAP:

1. "Moving" objects must be labeled with a fluorophore.
2. Equipment must be able to bleach a defined area.

FRAP detects:

- Diffusion of molecules
- Active movement of cell components
- Recycling of cell components

The modern fluorescence microscope can provide more information, further enhanced by the informatics instruments that are now available. Digital images combined with FRAP enable the acquisition of information at low light levels or at visually undetectable wavelengths. These technical improvements are now an integral part of the techniques discussed here. Several years ago, optical microscopy was purely a descriptive instrument, whereas now it represents the first step of a more detailed pathway. The microscope accomplishes this first step in conjunction with electronic detectors, image processors, and display devices that can be viewed as extensions of the imaging system.

Technique Description and Examples

The basic function of a fluorescence microscope is to irradiate specimens with the right wavelength and separate the weaker emitted fluorescence from the excitation light. Only the emission light should reach the eye, or detector, leading to fluorescent structures being displayed as a high-contrast color on a very dark (or black) background. The limits of detection are generally related to the darkness of the background and the excitation light, which is typically from several hundred thousand to a million times brighter than the emitted fluorescence. Photobleaching is the irreversible decomposition of the fluorescent molecules in the excited state because of their interaction with molecular oxygen before emission. Among very recent applications of the FRAP technique [104–110], we note investigations of chromatin mobility and structure [111, 112] and analysis of protozoan flagellar proteins [113].

Fluorescence Lifetime Imaging Microscopy (FLIM)

Fluorescence lifetime can be defined as the average time a molecule spends in its excited singlet state before spontaneous emission occurs. The fluorescence lifetime of a fluorophore can be described as the decrease in the number of excited fluorophores during the time following optical excitation with a very short light pulse. Generally, since the excited state of a fluorophore has a time interval between 1 and 20 ns, the excitation pulse must be about 100 ps to avoid excitation and emission coincident light. Fluorescence lifetime possesses some advantages over conventional fluorescence microscopy because each fluorescent dye has its own lifetime in the excited state. Thus, by detecting differences in lifetime, it is possible to distinguish dyes with overlapping fluorescent wavelengths or autofluorescence, which can be undistinguishable with conventional fluorescence microscopy based on spectral characteristics. In addition, fluorescence lifetime imaging microscopy (FLIM) finds its most significant applications in visualizing environmental changes of a probe in a living cell [97, 114]. As discussed previously, a fluorophore in the excited state possesses a higher dipolar moment that can be affected by solvent polarity changes due to ions, pH, and changes in its localization within the cell organelles or binding with other molecules [115–117]. Since the lifetime depends on the excited state, solvent change can change the lifetime of the fluorophore. In fact, the emission spectrum of the fluorophore also changes with solvent polarity; a maximum red shift is generally observed by increasing solvent polarity. However, this shift is generally smaller than the wavelength range of the band-pass emission filter. Furthermore, lifetime is independent of dye concentration, photobleaching, light scattering, and excitation light intensity; therefore, FLIM enables accurate ion concentration measurement and FRET analysis [118, 119].

Two methods of FLIM are used: the time–domain method and the frequency–domain method.

Frequency-Domain FLIM

In frequency–domain measurement, the sample is excited by a frequency sinusoidally modulated laser source (1–200 MHz). The phase and amplitude of the exciting light are measured; the lifetime of each fluorophore causes a unique phase shift and attenuation at a given frequency. The measurement may be taken either by a photomultiplier or using a CCD. However, this method, despite having a high temporal resolution, has limited ability to provide spatial information. Usually, FLIM instruments for frequency–domain methods are designed to operate at frequencies between 10 and 100 MHz, since most fluorochromes frequently used in biomedical research have lifetimes ranging from 1 to 10 ns [120].

Time–Domain FLIM

Time-resolved fluorescence takes advantage of high-speed pulsed lasers with picosecond pulses with fast recurrence rates and a high-speed gate image intensifier to acquire emitted photons. Emitted photons can be collected in two ways: time-correlated single photon counting (TCSPC) and the acquisition of a fixed number of photons (two to eight) in distinct time intervals using gated detection. In TCSPC, the elapsed time to reach the detector by the first photon after each pulse is monitored at a very high time resolution. A decay plot is obtained by recording the elapsed times of a large number of photons. In the other method, fluorescence intensity is monitored as a function of time by integrating the area under the curve describing the exponential decay at two distinct time intervals after pulse.

Frequency–domain FLIM was used by Bastiaens et al. [121] to measure the average fluorescence lifetimes of six GFP variants, which were found to range in value from 1.3 to 3.7 ns. The ability to distinguish fusion proteins labeled with different GFP variants gives the chance to obtain information from different proteins simultaneously in a single experiment using multi-labeling imaging of live cells. Sabatini et al. [115] measured cyclic adenosine monophosphate (cAMP)-dependent protein kinase A (PKA) activity in brain tissue in FRET–FLIM experiments using an A-kinase activity reporter (AKAR).

References

1. Parrilla E, Armengot M, Mata M, Sanchez-Vilchez JM, Cortijo J, Hueso JL, Riera J, Moratal D. Primary ciliary dyskinesia assessment by means of optical flow analysis of phase-contrast microscopy images. Comput Med Imaging Graph. 2014;38:163–70.

2. Kong L, Doona CJ, Setlow P, Li YQ. Monitoring rates and heterogeneity of high-pressure germination of bacillus spores by phase-contrast microscopy of individual spores. Appl Environ Microbiol. 2014;80:345–53.

3. Jaccard N, Griffin LD, Keser A, Macown RJ, Super A, Veraitch FS, Szita N. Automated method for the rapid and precise estimation of adherent cell culture characteristics from phase contrast microscopy images. Biotechnol Bioeng. 2014;111:504–17.

4. Thirusittampalam K, Hossain MJ, Ghita O, Whelan PF. A novel framework for cellular tracking and mitosis detection in dense phase contrast microscopy images. IEEE J Biomed Health Inform. 2013;17:642–53.

5. Steiger R, Bernet S, Ritsch-Marte M. Mapping of phase singularities with spiral phase contrast microscopy. Opt Express. 2013;21:16282–9.

6. Su H, Yin Z, Huh S, Kanade T. Cell segmentation in phase contrast microscopy images via semi-supervised classification over optics-related features. Med Image Anal. 2013;17:746–65.

7. Kong Z, Zhu X, Zhang S, Wu J, Luo Y. Phase contrast microscopy of living cells within the whole lens: spatial correlations and morphological dynamics. Mol Vis. 2012;18:2165–73.

8. Nejati Javaremi A, Unsworth CP, Graham ES. A cell derived active contour (CDAC) method for robust tracking in low frame rate, low contrast phase microscopy—an example: the human hNT astrocyte. PLoS One. 2013;8:e82883.

9. Rigaud S, Huang CH, Ahmed S, Lim JH, Racoceanu D. An analysis-synthesis approach for neurosphere modelisation under phase-contrast microscopy. Conf Proc IEEE Eng Med Biol Soc. 2013;2013:3989–92.

10. Liu A, Hao T, Gao Z, Su Y, Yang Z. Nonnegative mixed-norm convex optimization for mitotic cell detection in phase contrast microscopy. Comput Math Methods Med. 2013;2013:176272.

11. Huh S, Kanade T. Apoptosis detection for non-adherent cells in time-lapse phase contrast microscopy. Med Image Comput Comput Assist Interv. 2013;16:59–66.

12. Hooley EN, Tilley AJ, White JM, Ghiggino KP, Bell TD. Energy transfer in PPV-based conjugated polymers: a defocused widefield fluorescence microscopy study. Phys Chem Chem Phys. 2014;16:7108–14.

13. Juneau PM, Garnier A, Duchesne C. Selection and tuning of a fast and simple phase-contrast microscopy image segmentation algorithm for measuring myoblast growth kinetics in an automated manner. Microsc Microanal. 2013;19:855–66.

14. Huh S, Su H, Chen M, Kanade T. Efficient phase contrast microscopy restoration applied for muscle myotube detection. Med Image Comput Comput Assist Interv. 2013;16:420–7.

15. Kim J, An S, Ahn S, Kim B. Depth-variant deconvolution of 3D widefield fluorescence microscopy using the penalized maximum likelihood estimation method. Opt Express. 2013;21:27668–81.

16. Yin Z, Kanade T, Chen M. Understanding the phase contrast optics to restore artifact-free microscopy images for segmentation. Med Image Anal. 2012;16:1047–62.

17. Piper T, Piper J. Axial phase-darkfield-contrast (APDC), a new technique for variable optical contrasting in light microscopy. J Microsc. 2012;247:259–68.

18. Chatterjee S, Pavan Kumar Y. White light differential interference contrast microscope with a Sagnac interferometer. Appl Optics. 2014;53:296–300.

19. Chen J, Xu Y, Lv X, Lai X, Zeng S. Super-resolution differential interference contrast microscopy by structured illumination. Opt Express. 2013;21:112–21.

20. Chen J, Lv X, Zeng S. Doubling the resolution of spatial-light-modulator-based differential interference contrast microscopy by structured illumination. Opt Lett. 2013;38:3219–22.

21. Battle C, Lautscham L, Schmidt CF. Differential interference contrast microscopy using light-emitting diode illumination in conjunction with dual optical traps. Rev Sci Instrum. 2013;84:053703.

22. Kim M, Choi Y, Fang-Yen C, Sung Y, Kim K, Dasari RR, Feld MS, Choi W. Three-dimensional differential interference contrast microscopy using synthetic aperture imaging. J Biomed Opt. 2012;17:026003.

23. Luo Y, Sun W, Gu Y, Wang G, Fang N. Wavelength-dependent differential interference contrast microscopy: multiplexing detection using nonfluorescent nanoparticles. Anal Chem. 2010;82:6675–9.

24. Zhu Y, Shaked NT, Satterwhite LL, Wax A. Spectral-domain differential interference contrast microscopy. Opt Lett. 2011;36:430–2.

25. McIntyre TJ, Maurer C, Bernet S, Ritsch-Marte M. Differential interference contrast imaging using a spatial light modulator. Opt Lett. 2009;34:2988–90.

26. Yang X, Qin L, Liang W, Wang W, Tan J, Liang P, Xu J, Li S, Cui S. New bone formation and microstructure assessed by combination of confocal laser scanning microscopy and differential interference contrast microscopy. Calcif Tissue Int. 2014;94:338–47.

27. Oh J, Kim SH, Kim YJ, Lee H, Cho JH, Cho YH, Kim CK, Lee TJ, Lee S, Park KH, Yu HG, Lee HJ, Jun SC, Kim JH. Detection of retinitis pigmentosa by differential interference contrast microscopy. PLoS One. 2014;9:e97170.

28. McPhee CI, Zoriniants G, Langbein W, Borri P. Measuring the lamellarity of giant lipid vesicles with differential interference contrast microscopy. Biophys J. 2013;105:1414–20.

29. Baker-Groberg SM, Phillips KG, McCarty OJ. Quantification of volume, mass, and density of thrombus formation using brightfield and differential interference contrast microscopy. J Biomed Opt. 2013;18:16014.

30. Tsunoda M, Isailovic D, Yeung ES. Real-time three-dimensional imaging of cell division by differential interference contrast microscopy. J Microsc. 2008;232:207–11.

31. Yenjerla M, Lopus M, Wilson L. Analysis of dynamic instability of steady-state microtubules in vitro by video-enhanced differential interference contrast microscopy with an appendix by Emin Oroudjev. Methods Cell Biol. 2010;95:189–206.

32. Wolf DE. Fundamentals of fluorescence and fluorescence microscopy. Methods Cell Biol. 2013;114:69–97.

33. Webb DJ, Brown CM. Epi-fluorescence microscopy. Methods Mol Biol. 2013;931:29–59.

34. Renz M. Fluorescence microscopy-a historical and technical perspective. Cytometry A. 2013;83:767–79.

35. Basic Concepts in Fluorescence. http://micro.magnet.fsu.edu/primer/techniques/fluorescence/fluorescence intro.html

36. Fritzky L, Lagunoff D. Advanced methods in fluorescence microscopy. Anal Cell Pathol. 2013;36:5–17.

37. Luo W, He K, Xia T, Fang X. Single-molecule monitoring in living cells by use of fluorescence microscopy. Anal Bioanal Chem. 2013;405:43–9.

38. Tahir M, Khan A, Kaya H. Protein subcellular localization in human and hamster cell lines: employing local ternary patterns of fluorescence microscopy images. J Theor Biol. 2014;340:85–95.

39. Duheron V, Moreau M, Collin B, Sali W, Bernhard C, Goze C, Gautier T, Pais de Barros JP, Deckert V, Brunotte F, Lagrost L, Denat F. Dual labeling of lipopolysaccharides for SPECT-CT imaging and fluorescence microscopy. ACS Chem Biol. 2014;9:656–62.

40. Ujihara Y, Nakamura M, Miyazaki H, Wada S. Segmentation and morphometric analysis of cells from fluorescence microscopy images of cytoskeletons. Comput Math Methods Med. 2013;2013:381356.

41. Tapley A, Switz N, Reber C, Davis JL, Miller C, Matovu JB, Worodria W, Huang L, Fletcher DA, Cattamanchi A. Mobile digital fluorescence microscopy for diagnosis of tuberculosis. J Clin Microbiol. 2013;51:1774–8.

42. Scholz D, Fortsch J, Bockler S, Klecker T, Westermann B. Analyzing membrane dynamics with live cell fluorescence microscopy with a focus on yeast mitochondria. Methods Mol Biol. 2013;1033:275–83.

43. Yan Y, Petchprayoon C, Mao S, Marriott G. Reversible optical control of cyanine fluorescence in fixed and living cells: optical lock-in detection immuno-fluorescence imaging microscopy. Philos Trans R Soc Lond B Biol Sci. 2013;368:20120031.

44. Furia L, Pelicci PG, Faretta M. A computational platform for robotized fluorescence microscopy (I): high-content image-based cell-cycle analysis. Cytometry A. 2013;83:333–43.

45. Furia L, Pelicci PG, Faretta M. A computational platform for robotized fluorescence microscopy (II): DNA damage, replication, checkpoint activation, and cell cycle progression by high-content high-resolution multiparameter image-cytometry. Cytometry A. 2013;83:344–55.

46. Laser Scanning Confocal Microscopy. http://micro.magnet.fsu.edu/primer/techniques/confocal/index.html

47. Ragazzi M, Piana S, Longo C, Castagnetti F, Foroni M, Ferrari G, Gardini G, Pellacani G. Fluorescence confocal microscopy for pathologists. Mod Pathol. 2014;27:460–71.

48. Herberich G, Windoffer R, Leube RE, Aach T. Signal and noise modeling in confocal laser scanning fluorescence microscopy. Med Image Comput Comput Assist Interv. 2012;15:381–8.

49. Wu Y, Zinchuk V, Grossenbacher-Zinchuk O, Stefani E. Critical evaluation of quantitative colocalization analysis in confocal fluorescence microscopy. Interdiscip Sci. 2012;4:27–37.

50. Balestrieri ML, Giovane A, Milone L, Servillo L. Endothelial progenitor cells express PAF receptor and respond to PAF via Ca(2+)-dependent signaling. Biochim Biophys Acta. 2010;1801:1123–32.

51. Coxon FP. Fluorescence imaging of osteoclasts using confocal microscopy. Methods Mol Biol. 2012;816:401–24.

52. Kress A, Wang X, Ranchon H, Savatier J, Rigneault H, Ferrand P, Brasselet S. Mapping the local organization of cell membranes using excitation-polarization-resolved confocal fluorescence microscopy. Biophys J. 2013;105:127–36.

53. Feola A, Cimini A, Migliucci F, Iorio R, Zuchegna C, Rothenberger R, Cito L, Porcellini A, Unteregger G, Tombolini V, Giordano A, Di Domenico M. The inhibition of p85alphaPI3KSer83 phosphorylation prevents cell proliferation and invasion in prostate cancer cells. J Cell Biochem. 2013;114:2114–9.

54. Cosentino C, Di Domenico M, Porcellini A, Cuozzo C, De Gregorio G, Santillo MR, Agnese S, Di Stasio R, Feliciello A, Migliaccio A, Avvedimento EV. p85 regulatory subunit of PI3K mediates cAMP-PKA and estrogens biological effects on growth and survival. Oncogene. 2007;26:2095–103.

55. Longo C, Rajadhyaksha M, Ragazzi M, Nehal K, Gardini S, Moscarella E, Lallas A, Zalaudek I, Piana S, Argenziano G, Pellacani G. Evaluating ex vivo fluorescence confocal microscopy images of basal cell carcinomas in Mohs excised tissue. Br J Dermatol. 2014;171(3):561–70.

56. Dobbs JL, Ding H, Benveniste AP, Kuerer HM, Krishnamurthy S, Yang W, Richards-Kortum R. Feasibility of confocal fluorescence microscopy for real-time evaluation of neoplasia in fresh human breast tissue. J Biomed Opt. 2013;18:106016.

57. Bennassar A, Carrera C, Puig S, Vilalta A, Malvehy J. Fast evaluation of 69 basal cell carcinomas with ex vivo fluorescence confocal microscopy: criteria description, histopathological correlation, and inter-observer agreement. JAMA Dermatol. 2013;149:839–47.

58. De Gregorio G, Coppa A, Cosentino C, et al. The p85 regulatory subunit of PI3K mediates TSHcAMP-PKA growth and survival signals. Oncogene. 2007;26:2039–47.

59. Altomare DA, Testa JR. Perturbations of the AKT signaling pathway in human cancer. Oncogene. 2005;24:7455–64.

60. Vega FM, Fruhwirth G, Ng T, Ridley AJ. RhoA and RhoC have distinct roles in migration and invasion by acting through different targets. J Cell Biol. 2011;193:655–64.

61. Total Internal Reflection Fluorescence Microscopy. http://micro.magnet.fsu.edu/primer/techniques/fluorescence/tirf/tirfhome.html

62. Brunstein M, Teremetz M, Herault K, Tourain C, Oheim M. Eliminating unwanted far-field excitation in objective-type TIRF. Part I. Identifying sources of nonevanescent excitation light. Biophys J. 2014;106:1020–32.

63. Brunstein M, Herault K, Oheim M. Eliminating unwanted far-field excitation in objective-type TIRF. Part II. Combined evanescent-wave excitation and supercritical-angle fluorescence detection improves optical sectioning. Biophys J. 2014;106:1044–56.

64. Lane RS, Macpherson AN, Magennis SW. Signal enhancement in multiphoton TIRF microscopy by shaping of broadband femtosecond pulses. Opt Express. 2012;20:25948–59.

65. Johnson DS, Jaiswal JK, Simon S. Total internal reflection fluorescence (TIRF) microscopy illuminator for improved imaging of cell surface events. Curr Protoc Cytom. 2012;Chapter 12, Unit 12 29.

66. Liang L, Shen H, De Camilli P, Toomre DK, Duncan JS. An expectation maximization based method for subcellular particle tracking using multi-angle TIRF microscopy. Med Image Comput Comput Assist Interv. 2011;14:629–36.

67. Oheim M. Quantitative imaging of single-organelle and single-molecule dynamics near the plasma membrane using a combination of spinning TIRF and virtual supercritical-angle detection. Biomed Tech. 2012. doi:10.1515/bmt-2012-4565.

68. Charlton C, Gubala V, Gandhiraman RP, Wiechecki J, Le NC, Coyle C, Daniels S, Maccraith BD, Williams DE. TIRF microscopy as a screening method for non-specific binding on surfaces. J Colloid Interface Sci. 2011;354:405–9.

69. Parhamifar L, Moghimi SM. Total internal reflection fluorescence (TIRF) microscopy for real-time imaging of nanoparticle-cell plasma membrane interaction. Methods Mol Biol. 2012;906:473–82.

70. Loder MK, Tsuboi T, Rutter GA. Live-cell imaging of vesicle trafficking and divalent metal ions by total internal reflection fluorescence (TIRF) microscopy. Methods Mol Biol. 2013;950:13–26.

71. Leslie K, Galjart N. Going solo: measuring the motions of microtubules with an in vitro assay for TIRF microscopy. Methods Cell Biol. 2013;115:109–24.

72. Telley IA, Bieling P, Surrey T. Reconstitution and quantification of dynamic microtubule end tracking in vitro using TIRF microscopy. Methods Mol Biol. 2011;777:127–45.

73. Ross JA, Digman MA, Wang L, Gratton E, Albanesi JP, Jameson DM. Oligomerization state of dynamin 2 in cell membranes using TIRF and number and brightness analysis. Biophys J. 2011;100:L15–7.

74. Matz M, Schumacher K, Hatlapatka K, Lorenz D, Baumann K, Rustenbeck I. Observer-independent quantification of insulin granule exocytosis and pre-exocytotic mobility by TIRF microscopy. Microsc Microanal. 2014;20:206–18.

75. Akopova I, Tatur S, Grygorczyk M, Luchowski R, Gryczynski I, Gryczynski Z, Borejdo J, Grygorczyk R. Imaging exocytosis of ATP-containing vesicles with TIRF microscopy in lung epithelial A549 cells. Purinergic Signal. 2012;8:59–70.

76. Sidaway P, Teramoto N. L-type Ca^{2+} channel sparklets revealed by TIRF microscopy in mouse urinary bladder smooth muscle. PLoS One. 2014;9:e93803.

77. Ramachandran S, Arce FT, Patel NR, Quist AP, Cohen DA, Lal R. Structure and permeability of ion-channels by integrated AFM and waveguide TIRF microscopy. Sci Rep. 2014;4:4424.

78. Pietraszewska-Bogiel A, Gadella TW. FRET microscopy: from principle to routine technology in cell biology. J Microsc. 2011;241:111–8.

79. Sun Y, Wallrabe H, Seo SA, Periasamy A. FRET microscopy in 2010: the legacy of Theodor Forster on the 100th anniversary of his birth. Chemphyschem. 2011;12:462–74.

80. Giron MD, Salto R. From green to blue: site-directed mutagenesis of the green fluorescent protein to teach protein structure-function relationships. Biochem Mol Biol Educ. 2011;39:309–15.

81. Hoppe AD, Scott BL, Welliver TP, Straight SW, Swanson JA. N-way FRET microscopy of multiple

protein-protein interactions in live cells. PLoS One. 2013;8:e64760.

82. Kruger AC, Birkedal V. Single molecule FRET data analysis procedures for FRET efficiency determination: probing the conformations of nucleic acid structures. Methods. 2013;64:36–42.

83. Simkova E, Stanek D. Probing nucleic acid interactions and Pre-mRNA splicing by Forster resonance energy transfer (FRET) microscopy. Int J Mol Sci. 2012;13:14929–45.

84. Renciuk D, Zhou J, Beaurepaire L, Guedin A, Bourdoncle A, Mergny JL. A FRET-based screening assay for nucleic acid ligands. Methods. 2012;57:122–8.

85. Guo Q, He Y, Lu HP. Manipulating and probing enzymatic conformational fluctuations and enzyme-substrate interactions by single-molecule FRET-magnetic tweezers microscopy. Phys Chem Chem Phys. 2014;16(26):13052–8.

86. Canclini L, Wallrabe H, Di Paolo A, Kun A, Calliari A, Sotelo-Silveira JR, Sotelo JR. Association of Myosin Va and Schwann cells-derived RNA in mammal myelinated axons, analyzed by immunocytochemistry and confocal FRET microscopy. Methods. 2014;66:153–61.

87. Ziomkiewicz I, Loman A, Klement R, Fritsch C, Klymchenko AS, Bunt G, Jovin TM, Arndt-Jovin DJ. Dynamic conformational transitions of the EGF receptor in living mammalian cells determined by FRET and fluorescence lifetime imaging microscopy. Cytometry A. 2013;83:794–805.

88. Wallrabe H, Cai Y, Sun Y, Periasamy A, Luzes R, Fang X, Kan HM, Cameron LC, Schafer DA, Bloom GS. IQGAP1 interactome analysis by in vitro reconstitution and live cell 3-color FRET microscopy. Cytoskeleton. 2013;70:819–36.

89. Prasad S, Zeug A, Ponimaskin E. Analysis of receptor-receptor interaction by combined application of FRET and microscopy. Methods Cell Biol. 2013;117:243–65.

90. Grecco HE, Bastiaens PI. Quantifying cellular dynamics by fluorescence resonance energy transfer (FRET) microscopy. Curr Protoc Neurosci. 2013; Chapter 5, Unit 5 22.

91. Sprenger JU, Perera RK, Gotz KR, Nikolaev VO. FRET microscopy for real-time monitoring of signaling events in live cells using unimolecular biosensors. J Vis Exp. 2012;e4081.

92. Roberts SK, Tynan CJ, Winn M, Martin-Fernandez ML. Investigating extracellular in situ EGFR structure and conformational changes using FRET microscopy. Biochem Soc Trans. 2012;40:189–94.

93. Padilla-Parra S, Tramier M. FRET microscopy in the living cell: different approaches, strengths and weaknesses. Bioessays. 2012;34:369–76.

94. Ferrari ML, Gomez GA, Maccioni HJ. Spatial organization and stoichiometry of N-terminal domain-mediated glycosyltransferase complexes in Golgi

95. Day RN, Davidson MW. Fluorescent proteins for FRET microscopy: monitoring protein interactions in living cells. Bioessays. 2012;34:341–50.

96. Goncalves JT, Stuhmer W. Calmodulin interaction with hEAG1 visualized by FRET microscopy. PLoS One. 2010;5:e10873.

97. Ishikawa-Ankerhold HC, Ankerhold R, Drummen GP. Advanced fluorescence microscopy techniques–FRAP, FLIP, FLAP, FRET and FLIM. Molecules. 2012;17:4047–132.

98. Yang J, Kohler K, Davis DM, Burroughs NJ. An improved strip FRAP method for estimating diffusion coefficients: correcting for the degree of photobleaching. J Microsc. 2010;238:240–53.

99. Kang M, Day CA, DiBenedetto E, Kenworthy AK. A quantitative approach to analyze binding diffusion kinetics by confocal FRAP. Biophys J. 2010;99:2737–47.

100. Kang M, Day CA, Kenworthy AK, DiBenedetto E. Simplified equation to extract diffusion coefficients from confocal FRAP data. Traffic. 2012;13:1589–600.

101. Xiong R, Deschout H, Demeester J, De Smedt SC, Braeckmans K. Rectangle FRAP for measuring diffusion with a laser scanning microscope. Methods Mol Biol. 2014;1076:433–41.

102. Wachsmuth M. Molecular diffusion and binding analyzed with FRAP. Protoplasma. 2014;251:373–82.

103. Deschout H, Raemdonck K, Demeester J, De Smedt SC, Braeckmans K. FRAP in pharmaceutical research: practical guidelines and applications in drug delivery. Pharm Res. 2014;31:255–70.

104. Groeneweg FL, van Royen ME, Fenz S, Keizer VI, Geverts B, Prins J, de Kloet ER, Houtsmuller AB, Schmidt TS, Schaaf MJ. Quantitation of glucocorticoid receptor DNA-binding dynamics by single-molecule microscopy and FRAP. PLoS One. 2014;9: e90532.

105. Watanabe N, Yamashiro S, Vavylonis D, Kiuchi T. Molecular viewing of actin polymerizing actions and beyond: combination analysis of single-molecule speckle microscopy with modeling, FRAP and s-FDAP (sequential fluorescence decay after photoactivation). Dev Growth Differ. 2013;55:508–14.

106. Schneider K, Fuchs C, Dobay A, Rottach A, Qin W, Wolf P, Alvarez-Castro JM, Nalaskowski MM, Kremmer E, Schmid V, Leonhardt H, Schermelleh L. Dissection of cell cycle-dependent dynamics of Dnmt1 by FRAP and diffusion-coupled modeling. Nucleic Acids Res. 2013;41:4860–76.

107. Bougault C, Cueru L, Bariller J, Malbouyres M, Paumier A, Aszodi A, Berthier Y, Mallein-Gerin F, Trunfio-Sfarghiu AM. Alteration of cartilage mechanical properties in absence of beta1 integrins revealed by rheometry and FRAP analyses. J Biomech. 2013;46:1633–40.

108. Hardy LR. Fluorescence recovery after photobleaching (FRAP) with a focus on F-actin. Curr Protoc Neurosci. 2012;Chapter 2, Unit 2 17.

109. Day CA, Kraft LJ, Kang M, Kenworthy AK. Analysis of protein and lipid dynamics using confocal fluorescence recovery after photobleaching (FRAP). Curr Protoc Cytom. 2012;Chapter 2, Unit 2 19.

110. Aguila B, Simaan M, Laporte SA. Study of G protein-coupled receptor/beta-arrestin interactions within endosomes using FRAP. Methods Mol Biol. 2011;756:371–80.

111. Bošković A, Eid A, Pontabry J, Ishiuchi T, Spiegelhalter C, Raghu Ram EV, Meshorer E, Torres-Padilla ME. Higher chromatin mobility supports totipotency and precedes pluripotency in vivo. Genes Dev. 2014;28(10):1042–7.

112. Bernas T, Brutkowski W, Zarębski M, Dobrucki J. Spatial heterogeneity of dynamics of H1 linker histone. Eur Biophys J. 2014;43:287–300.

113. Subota I, Julkowska D, Vincensini L, Reeg N, Buisson J, Blisnick T, Huet D, Perrot S, Santi-Rocca J, Duchateau M, Hourdel V, Rousselle JC, Cayet N, Namane A, Chamot-Rooke J, Bastin P. Proteomic analysis of intact flagella of procyclic Trypanosoma brucei cells identifies novel flagellar proteins with unique sub-localisation and dynamics. Mol Cell Proteomics. 2014;13(7):1769–86.

114. Pande P, Jo JA. Automated analysis of fluorescence lifetime microscopy (FLIM) data based on the Laguerre deconvolution method. IEEE Trans BioMed Eng. 2011;58:172–81.

115. Chen Y, Saulnier JL, Yellen G, Sabatini BL. A PKA activity sensor for quantitative analysis of endogenous GPCR signaling via 2-photon FRET-FLIM imaging. Front Pharmacol. 2014;5:56.

116. Schmitt FJ, Thaa B, Junghans C, Vitali M, Veit M, Friedrich T. eGFP-pHsens as a highly sensitive fluorophore for cellular pH determination by fluorescence lifetime imaging microscopy (FLIM). Biochim Biophys Acta. 2014.

117. Paredes JM, Giron MD, Ruedas-Rama MJ, Orte A, Crovetto L, Talavera EM, Salto R, Alvarez-Pez JM. Real-time phosphate sensing in living cells using fluorescence lifetime imaging microscopy (FLIM). J Phys Chem B. 2013;117:8143–9.

118. Morton PE, Parsons M. Measuring FRET using time-resolved FLIM. Methods Mol Biol. 2011;769:403–13.

119. Oliveira AF, Yasuda R. An improved Ras sensor for highly sensitive and quantitative FRET-FLIM imaging. PloS one. 2013;8:e52874.

120. Schuermann KC, Grecco HE. flatFLIM: enhancing the dynamic range of frequency domain FLIM. Opt Express. 2012;20:20730–41.

121. Pepperkok R, Squire A, Geley S, Bastiaens PI. Simultaneous detection of multiple green fluorescent proteins in live cells by fluorescence lifetime imaging microscopy. Curr Biol. 1999;9:269–72.

Cytometry and Pathology

5

Virginia Tirino, Vincenzo Desiderio, Francesca Paino,
and Gianpaolo Papaccio

Introduction

Flow cytometry is a complex field that draws people from diverse scientific backgrounds. It is a technology that simultaneously measures and analyzes multiple physical characteristics of single particles, usually cells, as they flow in a fluid stream through a beam of light. The properties measured include a particle's relative size, relative granularity or internal complexity, and relative fluorescence intensity. These characteristics are determined using an optical-to-electronic coupling system that records how the cell or particle scatters incident laser light and emits fluorescence. Some flow cytometers are also equipped to identify and sort user-specified particles into collection vessels. High-performance cell sorters can routinely sort at rates of 70,000 cells per second. The strength of flow cytometers is that they can rapidly and quantitatively measure simultaneously multiple parameters of individual live cells and then isolate cells of interest. Additionally, the sensitivity and throughput rates achievable by high-performance commercial instruments enable the detection of extremely rare populations and events (frequencies below 10^{-6}), such as stem cells, dendritic cells, antigen-specific T cells, and genetic transfectants [1]. As a result, applications for flow cytometers continue to increase. In addition to traditional immunology and pathology applications involving particles such as lymphocytes, macrophages, monocytes, and tumor cells, flow cytometers are widely used in conjunction with fluorescence-based protein reporters, such as green fluorescent protein. In this context, flow cytometers can monitor both transfection efficiency and protein expression levels [2, 3]. In addition, interest is growing in the use of flow cytometers to screen cell- or bead-based combinatorial libraries [4]. Therefore, flow cytometry also enables the screening of protein libraries expressed in cells or displayed on the surface of bacteria or beads. A flow cytometer, for instance, can detect modulation of a signal transduction pathway by a particular small molecule and identify proteins with a particular binding specificity, enzymatic activity, expression level, and stability. Ongoing development efforts in the flow cytometry industry are aimed at automation and laboratory integration. Input/output robotics, pushbutton operations, and automated sample preparation will increase throughput rates and make the technology more accessible to a wider user base, as new fluorescent dyes and creative screening approaches expand applications into the proteomic field. Eventually, software advances will seamlessly network instruments into comprehensive analytical and

V. Tirino (✉) • V. Desiderio • F. Paino • G. Papaccio
Dipartimento di Medicina Sperimentale, Sezione di
Biotecnologie, Istologia Medica e Biologia Molecolare,
Seconda Università degli Studi di Napoli, Napoli, Italy
e-mail: virginia.tirino@unina2.it

© Springer Science+Business Media New York 2016
F.M. Sacerdoti et al. (eds.), *Advanced Imaging Techniques in Clinical Pathology*,
Current Clinical Pathology, DOI 10.1007/978-1-4939-3469-0_5

diagnostic systems, and the industry may marry its technology with imaging and microfluidics.

Scope

In this chapter, the main aspects of flow cytometry as applied to pathology are described: a brief history of cytometry, the characteristics of cells suitable for flow cytometry, methods used to identify cell phenotypes, cell sorting, cell cycle analyses, and data analyses. This chapter can be read as a self-contained brief of the field of flow cytometry.

Historical Background

The evolution of flow cytometry can be divided into four distinct phases:

1. The development of microscopy
2. The development of dye chemistry
3. The development of electronics
4. The development of computers

All these produced instruments coincident with global biomedical need.

In the sixteenth century, Leeuwenhoek built the first microscope to visualize protozoa and bacteria and can thus be considered the father of cytometry. By 1742, Lomonosov had described the method for producing dark-field illumination and performed light scatter measurements. Light was the sole means of illumination until 1904, when Kolher developed a microscope with an ultraviolet (UV) light source. Essentially, all further developments centered on the microscope until 1934, when Moldavan [5] described a photoelectric technique for counting cells flowing through a capillary tube, and flow cytometry was born. In 1938, Caspersson built a rudimentary flow cytometer to measure cell properties in the ultraviolet and visible regions. Crosland and Tylor developed a blood cell counter using the sheath flow principle, light scatter, and dark-field illumination in 1940. Following work by various researchers in

subsequent decades to develop instruments to count particles in suspension [6–9], Kamentsky and Melamed [10, 11] implemented a design in 1965 and 1967 to produce a microscope-based flow cytometer for detecting light signals to distinguish abnormal cells in a cervical sample. Following this, the work of Fulwyler [12], Dittrich and Göhde [13], Van Dilla et al. [14], and Hulett et al. [15] led to significant changes and resulted in a cytometer that largely resembled those of today. Like modern cytometers, a flow cytometer in 1969 in no way resembled a microscope but was still based on Moldavan's prototype and on the Kamentsky instrument in that it illuminated cells as they progressed in single file in front of a beam of light, and it used photodetectors to detect the signals that came from the cells [15–18]. Even today, the definition of a flow cytometer involves an instrument that illuminates cells as they flow individually in front of a light source and then detects and correlates the signals from those cells as a result of that illumination.

Stains were required to enhance the visibility of prokaryotic and eukaryotic material under the microscope. The development of these stains was driven by the absorptive dye chemistry needed in the textile industry after 1850. Malachowski and Romanowsky [19, 20] used acidic and basic dyes, which gave rise to the Giemsa, Leishman, MacNeal, and Wright stains used for identifying parasites in blood cells and hematopoietic cells. Fluorescent dyes did not appear until the 1880s, when Paul Ehrlich [21] synthesized and used fluorescein. He also pioneered the use of mixtures of acidic and basic dyes to resolve the internal structure of leukocytes. DNA dyes were first used in 1900, but the introduction of flow cytometry drove the development of several new dyes in the late 1960s and 1970s, and the measurement of DNA content became one of the first major applications of flow cytometry. Dittrich and Göhde [22] first used ethidium bromide in 1969, Crissman and Steinkamp [23] introduced propidium iodide in 1973, and Crissman and Tobey [24] used mithramycin in 1974. In 1976, Latt and Stetten [25] introduced the Hoechst dyes, and a year later Stöhr et al. [26] used 4',6-

diamidino-2-phenylindole) (DAPI). All of these dyes are commonly used in modern flow cytometry. In parallel, in 1940, Coons et al. [27] used antipneumococcal antibodies conjugated with anthracene to detect microorganisms in tissues. By 1950, they were using antibodies conjugated with fluorescein isothiocyanate (FITC), and immunophenotyping was born. Immunophenotyping allowed for the labeling of specific cell membrane proteins on cells, predominately leukocytes. Instead of relying on morphology, scientists could now identify cells by their unique repertoire of membrane proteins. In 1974, Kano et al. [28] introduced the process of producing monoclonal antibodies.

Meanwhile, development was ongoing in the electronics industry. By 1945, the photomultiplier tube (PMT) had been developed to detect photons and convert them to electrical pulses. Amplifiers and analog-to-digital converters were also developed. In 1949, Wallace Coulter [29] patented the first non-optical electronic blood cell counter; by the 1950s, the realization that automated cytology might be most useful in clinical diagnosis began to permeate academic medical institutions. The ability to electronically count blood cells more accurately and faster than with a hemocytometer started the revolution towards automation. The first Model A Coulter counter was introduced in 1957, primarily to count erythrocytes and leukocytes from blood; Model B was introduced 4 years later. This device could also provide the size distribution of these cells. The disadvantage of the Coulter Counter was that it could not identify what was being counted. This led to the need for an automated microscopic identification process. To accomplish this, computers, which had recently been introduced, and the concomitant software, were required. Two different groups emerged to tackle this problem. Marylou Ingram (a hematologist at the University of Rochester) and Kendall Preston [30] (a biomedical engineer at Perkin–Elmer) together built the first cytoanalyzer, a microscope-based instrument, to automate the microscopic identification of leukocytes in stained smears. At the same time,

another group, Mortimer Mendelssohn, and Judith Prewitt [31], began studies to extend the image analysis of cells using an automated instrument called a "CYDAC". This was the first example of automated image cytometry. Cells could now flow through an orifice and be counted; they could also be stained and identified microscopically in a somewhat automated fashion.

Modern flow cytometry began when Fulwyler [32], at the US Los Alamos National Laboratories, built a cell sorter using the main Coulter cell size and the electrostatic charging of the droplets to order. Then, Dittrich and Göhde [22] developed the impulse cytophotometer (ICP), also known as the "Phywe." Cells were introduced into a flowing sheath stream located under a high-power microscope objective that provided measures of scatter and fluorescence detection. Mullaney and Dean [33] introduced multiparametric flow cytometry, combining the measurement of volume, light scatter, and fluorescence in a single instrument. By the mid-1970s, flow cytometers had entered the market, and Leonard Herzenberg [34] coined the term "fluorescence activated cell sorter," or "FACS," revolutionizing immunology and cancer biology. In the early 1980s, interest in immunophenotyping grew with the discovery of AIDS. The first monoclonal antibodies identified membrane proteins such as CD3, CD4, and CD8 expressed by T lymphocytes. The first major clinical application of immunophenotyping using flow cytometry was in the treatment of AIDS. With this development, and the ability to measure DNA content, flow cytometry became the important and primary approach to automated cell analysis in clinical applications. These applications included ploidy and S-phase fraction measurement in solid tumors, diagnosis and follow-up of hematopoietic malignancies and paroxysmal nocturnal hemoglobinuria (PNH), and monitoring of transplant rejection and hematopoietic regeneration. Whereas immunophenotyping initially focused on the measurement of membrane markers on the cells, researchers soon found that intracellular markers could also be measured. With its ability to identify a cell population from membrane markers and simultaneously determine the function of the cell, the power of flow cytometry was quickly realized. Another application launched by Stubblefield et al. [35] in Los Alamos and van den Engh et al. [36] at the Lawrence Livermore National Laboratory was chromosome staining and sorting for DNA cloning to produce chromosome-specific sequences. This new application led to the construction of the first high-speed cell sorter to classify each human chromosome. This project, supported by the US Department of Energy, was the first step in the Human Genome Project. Hence, since a very slow start in the seventeenth century, the development of chemical dyes, the electronics industry, the computer, and the production of monoclonal antibodies have all come together to produce the rapidly expanding field of flow cytometry. No other technology has been developed that can quickly measure the related properties of basic cells.

Techniques

The word "cytometer" itself is derived from two Greek words, "κιτοζ," meaning container, receptacle, or body (taken in modern formations to mean cell), and "μετρον," meaning measure. Cytometers measure particles. "Particle" can be used as a more general term for any of the objects flowing through a flow cytometer. "Event" is used to indicate anything that has been interpreted by the instrument, correctly or incorrectly, to be a single particle. For example, if the cytometer is not quick enough, two particles close together may actually be detected as one event. Because most of the particles sent through cytometers and detected as events are in fact single cells, the words are used somewhat interchangeably.

Flow Cytometry and Particles/Events

Because flow cytometry is a technique for the analysis of individual particles, a flow cytometrist must begin by obtaining a suspension of particles. Historically, the particles analyzed by flow cytometry were often cells from blood; they are ideally suited for this technique because they exist as single cells and require no manipulation before cytometric analysis. Cultured cells or cell lines have also proven suitable, although adherent cells require some treatment to remove them from the surface on which they are grown. More recently, bacteria [37, 38], sperm [39, 40], and plankton [41] have been analyzed. Flow techniques have also been used to analyze individual particles that are not cells (e.g., viruses [42], nuclei [43], chromosomes [44], DNA fragments [45], and latex beads [46]). In addition, cells that do not occur as single particles can be made suitable for flow cytometric analysis using mechanical disruption or enzymatic digestion; tissues can be disaggregated into individual cells, and these can be run through a flow cytometer. The advantage of a method that analyzes single cells is that cells can be scanned rapidly (500 to >5000 per second), and the individual characteristics of a large number of cells can be enumerated, correlated, and summarized. The disadvantage of a single-cell technique is that cells that do not occur as individual particles must be disaggregated; when tissues are disaggregated for analysis, some of the characteristics of the individual cells can be altered and all information about tissue architecture and cell distribution is lost. Therefore, when the cell suspension used for cytometric analyses derives from cell culture or fresh biopsy, careful evaluation of the resulting data is necessary.

Immunophenotyping

Immunophenotyping of biological samples refers to the use of immunological tools (e.g., monoclonal and/or polyclonal antibodies) for the specific detection of antigens, most frequently from proteins, expressed by cells localized either on their surface or inside them. Flow cytometry is a sensitive technique currently employed by pathologists, especially for quantitative and qualitative evaluation of hematopoietic cells [46].

In a clinical setting, the main purpose of flow cytometric analysis is to identify abnormal cells by defining their immunophenotypic characteristics. To accomplish this task, multiparameter analysis represents a reliable approach that integrates the information provided by forward scatter (FSC) and side scatter (SSC) with multiple fluorescence parameters. Thus, the cell size and internal complexity as well as the simultaneous expression of three to four or more different cell antigens are evaluated and used to outline distinct cell populations [47]. Importantly, multiparameter analysis permits the detection of abnormal cells that occur at a very low frequency in the context of normal populations, such as in the case of minimal residual disease [48]. Multicolor flow cytometry is currently used by many laboratories for the analysis of leukemia and lymphoma, although technology is moving rapidly towards more complex types of analysis, employing six or more fluorescence parameters. In multicolor analysis, a widely used strategy for the gating of lymphocytes is based on CD45 expression and SSC characteristics [49]. This approach permits the analysis of aged samples with a better lymphocyte recovery than FCS vs. SSC gating. Therefore, gating via CD45/ SSC represents the strategy of choice for immunophenotyping blood lymphocyte subsets, for example, monitoring CD4 counts in patients with AIDS. The staging of human immunodeficiency virus (HIV) infection based on the enumeration of the absolute and relative CD4+ T-cell counts in peripheral blood probably represents the most extended and recognized clinical application of flow cytometry. Gating via CD45/SSC strategy is also being applied successfully in the analysis of many lymphoid malignancies detected in blood, bone marrow, and lymph nodes [50]. Specific immunophenotypic profiles have been established for several lymphoid neoplasms [51–53]. The abnormal profiles are compared with the pattern of cell marker expression normally seen in the organ/tissue being examined, and a diagnostic interpretation is made. While the normal reference ranges for differentiation antigens expressed by lymphoid cells from peripheral blood, bone marrow, and lymph nodes are well established, immunophenotyping is also currently a primary diagnostic tool for the study of individuals suspected of PNH, systemic mastocytosis (SM), primary thrombocytopathies, and immunodeficiencies. In all four disease groups, genetic abnormalities carried by the clonal hematopoietic cells are translated into changes in the phenotype and distribution of specific populations of hematopoietic cells. Such phenotypic changes are closely associated with specific underlying genetic abnormalities and can be easily and reproducibly identified with flow cytometry immunophenotyping. Although immunophenotyping does not allow a final diagnosis of most primary immunodeficiencies, it has great value as a screening tool. It is well established for that an association exists between the distribution of different populations of peripheral blood lymphocytes, their immunophenotype, and the underlying genetic defect. More detailed knowledge of the exact genetic lesions present in patients with primary immune deficiencies has largely contributed to expanding the utility of immunophenotyping in the diagnosis of this heterogeneous group of disorders.

Over the last decade, the application of flow cytometry immunophenotyping in transplantation has increased in terms of both hematopoietic tissues and solid organs. The most widely used example is the flow cytometry enumeration of CD34+ hematopoietic progenitors to control the quality of biological products obtained for hematopoietic transplantation. It is well established that the total number of CD34 +CD45dim hematopoietic progenitors given in a transplant is the most powerful indicator of the outcome of the graft, and flow cytometry immunophenotyping is the method of choice for counting CD34 cells. Another clinically relevant application of immunophenotyping in transplantation is the so-called flow cytometry crossmatch. The goal of this assay is to identify the presence of anti-human leukocyte antigen (HLA) antibodies, quantify their titer, and determine their specificities in the serum of the donor prior to an allogenic transplant. Although flow cytometry cross-match initially used cellular-based assays, in recent years they have been combined with multiplexed bead arrays that allow routine determination of anti-HLA antibody specificities. The use of cytometry for immunophenotyping has the advantage of quick multiparametric analysis of a very large number of cells (20,000–50,000) and a better statistical representation of the population of interest. The choice of the appropriate antibody combinations, gating strategy, and multiparametric analysis plays a key role in diagnosis. Cytometric analysis offers another advantage over other techniques: dual and triple markers can be applied to detect co-expression of two or three antigens on the same cell. Flow cytometry also has the ability to precisely detect immunoglobulin light chain expression and therefore assess the monoclonality of lymphoid populations. However, its major disadvantage lies in its need for mono-dispersed cell suspensions: fresh specimens are required to maintain viability and avoid loss of antigenicity through tissue fixation. Samples must be immediately suspended in chilled nutritional medium after surgical excision, followed by processing of fresh tissue within minutes or only a few hours. In addition, the information provided about the morphology and localization of a given molecule inside a cell is limited. On the other hand, immunohisto-chemistry (IHC) on paraffin-embedded tissue is limited by poor antigen preservation and difficulties in defining antigens that are restricted to cell surfaces; these are lost through fixation and include the majority of lymphoid markers. Sufficient antibodies have been developed for the identification of B- and T-cell populations on paraffin-embedded tissue. However, immuno-globulin light chains are not reliably demonstrated on cell surfaces by this method [54]. It has been reported that IHC does not usually provide clear evidence of surface light chain restriction due to the large amount of background immunoglobulin in the interstitial spaces of tissues, which obscures the relatively weak monoclonal immunoglobulins on the surface of B cells. However, flow cytometry is also more sensitive than molecular techniques (reverse transcription polymerase chain reaction [RT-PCR], quantitative RT-PCR [Q-RT-PCR]) as there is no possibility of sample contamination by non-neoplastic cells. In addition, complementary DNA (c-DNA) arrays are costly and tedious sophisticated lengthy tests that can only be performed in specialized laboratories and requires significant experience and a special software system. The possibilities for immunophe-notyping by flow cytometry are almost infinite in both clinical and research applications. In general, cells stained with antibodies may be used to identify, count, and characterize any type of individual cell or subcellular component. Many of the applications for immunophenotyping are of great clinical utility, mainly in the area of hematology and immunology.

Procedures

Immunophenotyping techniques measure antigen expression by flow cytometry. Traditionally, these techniques have been divided into two major methods: (1) direct immunofluorescence staining and (2) indirect immunofluorescence staining. The first is obtained when the antigen/antibody reaction is detected with an antibody directly coupled to a fluorochrome; the second requires the use of a secondary anti-immunoglobulin antibody conjugated to a fluorochrome. Given the complexity of performing multiple stains with indirect immunofluorescence methods, the use of these techniques is currently restricted almost exclusively to single antigen stains. Direct immunofluorescence is the preferred method for multicolor antibody/antigen reactions. Usually, the optimal sample preparation technique depends on the type of specimen and the cells of interest, the antigens and their distribution in the sample, the localization of the antigens in the cell, and the information to be obtained. The main steps to obtaining direct staining for immunophenotyping are as follows:

- Disaggregation of solid tissue or detachment of cells derived from cell culture
- Washing with PBS
- Adding the antibody on pellet

- Incubation, usually for 30 min at 4 °C in the dark
- Washing with PBS
- Acquisition and analysis with flow cytometry

Depending on the characteristics of the cells, specific changes in sample preparation techniques may also be required. For example, for the staining of non-nucleated red cells, the lysing steps should be eliminated, and quenching reagents (e.g., crystal violet) may be required for optimal immunophenotyping of highly autofluorescent cells. Another technique that requires modification of the immunofluorescence protocols is the staining of intracellular antigens: appropriate fixation and permeabilization protocols should be used prior to staining.

Finally, the type of information desired may also affect the exact sample preparation protocol to be applied. In fact, if immunophenotyping is used to count the number of cells present in a given volume of sample, washing steps and solutions that may damage the sample cells should be eliminated to avoid significant cell loss. Overall, variables that determine the most appropriate sample preparation protocol also determine the most appropriate instrument settings during data acquisition and the number of events that should be measured in the flow cytometer. It is well established that identification of a cell population requires a minimum of between 13 and 15 homogenous events, while reaching an acceptable coefficient of variation (10 %) for the enumeration of a cell population requires that a minimum of 100 cells of interest are analyzed. Table 5.1 shows the main variables that can affect the detection of antigen expression by flow cytometry.

DNA Measurement

In recent years, flow cytometry has been recognized as a useful, rapid, and novel method to determine—efficiently, reproducibly, and at lower costs per sample—the relative nuclear DNA content and ploidy level of cells. This technology has also been used to isolate cell population with different DNA content. On the consequence, after immunofluorescence, DNA analysis is the second most important application of flow cytometry. DNA measurement is very important because we obtain two main information: (1) ploidy, relevant in tumors, and (2) distribution of cells in phases of cell cycle. DNA is a molecule that carries most of the genetic instructions used in the growth, development, functioning and reproduction of all known living organisms. It is composed of bases that form two strands arranged as double helix. Being mainly involved in cell life in terms of reproduction, growth and death and tumor development, DNA study has aroused enormous interest to research and clinical cytometrists. To perform DNA analyses, fluorescent probes such as propidium iodide, DRAQ5 (a Vybrant DyeCycle compound) or the bis-benzimidazole, Hoechst 33342, can be used. Usually, fluorescent signal is proportional to the DNA amount in the nucleus identifying strong gains or losses in DNA content. Interestingly, it is the study of abnormal DNA content, defined as "DNA content aneuploidy," especially in tumors; although, some benign conditions may be aneuploid [55–60]. In several types of tumors, DNA aneuplody is correlated with a bad prognosis, but it may be associated with improved survival in rhabdo myosarcoma, neuroblastoma, multiple myeloma,

Table 5.1 List of the main variables in analyzing antigen expression in immunophenotyping

Monoclonal antibody reagents	Sample preparation	Fluorescence measurements
Affinity	Time	Nozzle size
Avidity	Temperature	Fluorescence detectors
Concentration	pH	Speed of analyses
Fluorochrome	Lysing solution	Instrument settings
Immunoglobulin isotype	Washing steps/autofluorescence	Compensation

and childhood acute lymphoblastic leukemia (ALL) [61–64]. For example, in ALL, hypodiploid tumors, myedisplastic syndromes, DNA hypodiploid content lead to a poor prognosis. On the contrary, DNA hyperdiploid content in ALL have a better prognosis [64]. Regarding hematologic tumors, data are discordant on the independent prognostic value of DNA content analyses.

DNA Probes

Before we focus on the measurement of DNA content, we provide a small prompt on the cell cycle. It is usually subdivided in three phases: the G_0G_1, S, and G_2M phases of the cell cycle, as shown in Fig. 5.1.

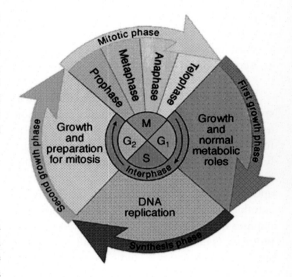

Fig. 5.1 Main phases of the cell cycle

G_0 (gap) is a phase in which cells are quiescent and not undergoing cell division.

G_1 is the phase in which cells are preparing to move through cell division and start to synthesize the factors involved in S phase. Both in G_0 and G_1, the DNA content is 2n. Therefore, both phases are indistinguishable from each other using a single DNA probe.

S (synthesis) is the phase in which the synthesis of DNA occurs. Therefore the DNA content ranges from 2n to 4n.

G_2 is the phase where the cells start to synthesize all components involved in M phase.

M (mitosis) is the phase in which it has the physical division of the mother cell with the formation of two daughter cells. Again, these two phases are indistinguishable from each other by the flow cytometer with a single DNA probe because the DNS content is 4n.

In order to measure the DNA content by flow cytometry, it is necessary to stain the nucleic acids using specific fluorescent probes. The bond between DNA and probe is not as strong as that of the antibody with its antigen. Therefore, it is important to establish the specific concentration of probes that must be used for DNA staining in cytometry, and samples are not washed after staining also because the unbound dye does not emit fluorescence. There are two main classes of DNA probes: (1) intercalating agents and (2) agents binding specifically to DNA bases. Intercalating agents usually intercalate between the bases in double-stranded nucleic acids, DNA or RNA. Therefore, these probes can also stain RNA and not only DNA. On the consequence, RNA must be eliminated using RNase that is added to staining solution. The advantage of these dyes is they are stoichiometric. Hence, the number of molecules of dye bound to DNA is equivalent to the number of DNA molecules. As a result, the amount of emitted light is proportional to the amount of bound dye that, in turn, is equivalent to DNA amount. Usually, intecalating probes belong to the family of phenanthridiniums and include propidium iodide and ethidium bromide. They are excite with ultraviolet or blue laser and emit in red spectrum. The Table 5.2 shows the properties of some mainly used DNA probes. The most widely used dye is propidium iodide (PI), which emits in red spectrum and is excited at 488 nm with blue laser. Unfortunately, the PI shows two disadvantages. First, PI stains both the DNA and double-stranded RNA. Therefore, the cells must be treated with RNase. Second, it is excluded by the plasma membrane. On the consequence, the cells must be fixed and, then, permeabilized. Subsequently, the probe can be added to cell preparation. Appropriate protocols for PI staining are found in Ormerod [65] and Darzynkiewicz [66]. For fixation, usually, 70 % ethanol is used or cells are suspended in a buffer containing a detergent [67]. The Fig. 5.2 shows a typical DNA histogram obtained using PI staining. The stromal population of normal diploid cells is usually not cycling. To analyze the DNA content, the fluorescence must be read using a linear scale. This strategy allows to determine quickly DNA index values. The second class of DNA probes includes dyes that bind preferentially to adenine-thymine (A-T) regions of DNA. This stain binds into the minor groove of DNA and exhibits distinct fluorescence emission spectra that are dependent on dye: base pair ratios. DAPI, either DRAQ5 (a Vybrant DyeCycle compound) or the bis-benzimidazole, Hoechst 3334,2 belong to this class of probes. DAPI and Hoechst3342 show an emission at 358 nm and 346 nm, respectively. Their emission is 461 nm. Therefore it is necessary an ultraviolet (UV) or violet laser. DRAQ5 probe is excited with 488 or 633 nm laser and its emission is 680 nm. In addition, DAPI is used for cells that must be fixed and permeabilized, whereas Hoechst33342 and DRAQ5 are vital probes, thus the cells must not be fixed. Independently of the dye used, it is necessary to perform preliminary assays to evaluate and determine the correct and specific times of incubation and dye concentration to obtain a satisfactory DNA histogram. Times and concentration are specific for each type of cells. In clinic diagnosis, DNA is extracted starting from sections of 50 μm thick of paraffin embedded tissues. The paraffin is removed, and the nuclei are extracted by treatment with pepsin [68]. The quality of the histograms can be very good, and depends on especially the way in which the tissue was initially handled. A strategy commonly used is to incubate tissue sections at 80 °C before treating with pepsin [69].

Table 5.2 Main DNA probes used in cytometry

Probe	Maximum excitation (nm)	Laser (nm)	Maximum emission (nm)	Features
Propidium Iodide	535	Blue (488)	623	Intercalating agent—not vital dye
Hoechst 33342	350	UV (355)	461	Bind strongly to A-T-rich regions in DNA—vital dye
DAPI	358	UV (355)	461	Bind strongly to A-T-rich regions in DNA—not vital dye
DRAQ5	650	Blue (488) or red (633)	680	Bind strongly to A-T-rich regions in DNA—vital dye

Fig. 5.2 This single-parameter histogram shows fluorescence on a linear scale along the x-axis, with number of events up the y-axis

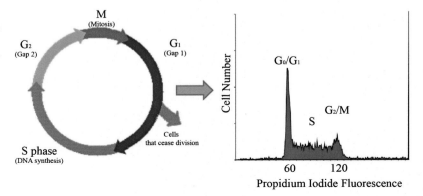

Ploidy

The ploidy of a cell is an indication of the number of chromosomes in that cell. Each species has a different ploidy value. There can also be variations within an individual population because of mutations, natural multiploidy (plants), certain diseases, and apoptosis. The number of chromosomes in a tumor is frequently greater than $2n$ (hyperdiploid) and sometimes less (hypodiploid). An abnormal number of chromosomes is called aneuploidy and is reflected by a change in the amount of DNA. The flow cytometrist tries to define these different ploidy levels and may use a series of definitions and terms, as reported in Table 5.3.

Therefore, when aneuploidy is measured as a change in DNA content, as opposed to a change in the number of chromosomes, it should be referred to as DNA aneuploidy. The DNA content of a tumor may be expressed as the DNA index (DI), defined as the ratio between the DNA content of a tumor cell and that of a normal diploid cell; Fig. 5.3 provides an example.

The quality of a DNA histogram is estimated from the width of the peak of DNA from cells in G1 of the cycle. This is measured by the coefficient of variation (CV) across the peak and is calculated from the standard deviation (SD).

The smaller the CV of the peaks in the DNA histogram, the more accurate the measurement of ploidy and the better the estimation of the percentage of cells in the different compartments of the cell cycle. It is essential that any unnecessary broadening of the peaks because of misalignment of the instrument should be eliminated. It is possible to obtain CVs as low as 1 %, although the best CV may be closer to 2 % in aneuploid tumors and cultured cells because of the heterogeneity of the DNA content. The number of clumps and the amount of debris present are also important factors. The key elements in obtaining a high-quality histogram are sample preparation, instrument alignment, and data analysis. The object of sample preparation is to obtain single cells (or nuclei) with the minimum of debris and clumps. When staining fixed cells with propidium iodide, sufficient time must be allowed for the RNase to remove all double-stranded RNA. If the cells have been fixed, leaving them overnight at 4 °C will often improve the histogram. If the cell (or nuclei) concentration is high, there should be sufficient dye present to maintain stoichiometric binding. The performance of the instrument should be checked daily using fluorescent beads of known CV, which can be purchased from several manufacturers. The CV and the peak channel number for a standard set of conditions (laser power, PMT voltage, and gain) should be recorded. If these fall outside predetermined limits (e.g., 2 % CV), action should be taken to restore the instrument's performance. Check that the flow rate has not been accidentally set too high; check there is no partial blockage of the flow cell; and, if possible (with a conventional cell sorter), realign the instrument.

If realignment is not possible (most bench-top instruments), call the service engineer. Any perturbation of the sample stream in the cytometer will increase the CV, so the concentration of cells or nuclei should be kept high (between 5×10^5 and 2×10^6/ml) and the flow rate low. The DNA histogram should be displayed on a linear scale.

Table 5.3 Definitions to indicate the ploidy value

Definitions	DNA content
Diploid	The normal (euploid) $2n$ number of chromosomes. This is the number of chromosomes in a somatic cell for a particular species
Haploid	Half the normal $2n$ number of chromosomes, or $1n$. This is the number of chromosomes in a gamete or germ cell (sperm/egg). Again, this is species dependent
Hyperdiploid	More than the normal $2n$ number of chromosomes
Hypodiploid	Less than the normal $2n$ number of chromosomes
Tetraploid	Double the normal $2n$ number of chromosomes, or $4n$
Aneuploid	An abnormal number of chromosomes

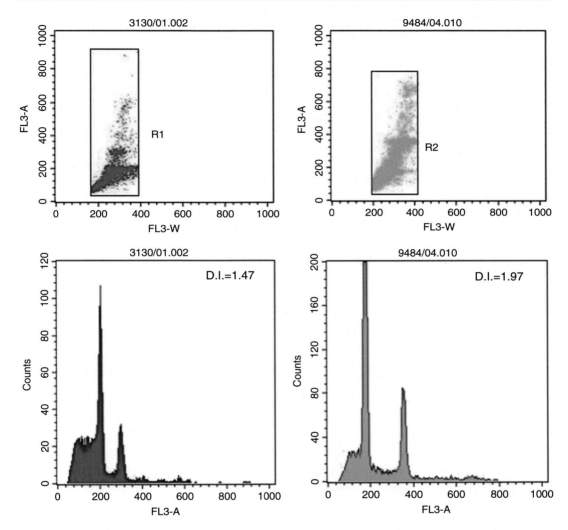

Fig. 5.3 DNA histograms from two endometrial carcinomas. Cells stained with propidium iodide (PI). DNA index (DI) values indicate samples with aneuploidy. Specifically, DNA content is hyperdiploid

Double Discrimination

One problem that must be overcome when obtaining results for DNA analysis is the exclusion of clumps of cells. On a flow cytometer, two cells stuck together may register as a single event, known as a doublet. If each of those two cells is diploid $(2n)$, seen as one event, they have 4n DNA. In other words, they have the same amount of DNA as a tetraploid cell (G0G1) or a normal cell that is about to divide (G2M). To add to the confusion, further peaks may exist for three or more cells stuck together. The doublet problem is resolved by employing a doublet discrimination gate based on the characteristics of fluorescence height, fluorescence area, and signal width. Fluorescence height is the maximum fluorescence given out by each cell as it travels through the laser beam; fluorescence area is the total amount of fluorescence emitted during the same journey; and signal width is the time a cell takes to pass through the laser beam. These characteristics differ between a cell that is about to divide and two cells that are stuck together.

A dividing cell does not double its membrane and cytoplasmic size and therefore passes through the laser beam more quickly than two cells stuck together. In other words, it has a smaller width signal or a bigger height signal but the same area as two cells stuck together. Also, all of the DNA in the dividing cell is grouped together in one nucleus and consequently gives off a greater intensity of emitted fluorescence than the DNA in two cells that are stuck together. Thus, a doublet, which has two nuclei separated by cytoplasm, emits a lower-intensity signal over a longer period. This appears as a greater width signal and lower height signal, with the same area. These differences can be seen on histograms of FL3-Area vs. FL3-Width (as shown in Fig. 5.3) or FL3-Area vs. FL3 Height, allowing the generation of gates to exclude doublets from sample analysis for both diploid and aneuploid cells.

Data Analysis and Reporting of the Cell Cycle Phases

There is obviously considerable overlap between early S phase and G1 and between late S phase and G2M because of the broadening of the distribution caused by variability in the staining of the cells as well as instrumental variability. The problem with analysis of a DNA histogram is finding a model to reliably estimate the extent of the overlap. The variety of approaches for modeling the cell cycle phases have been summarized by Rabinovitch [70]. The most rigorous algorithm is probably the polynomial method of Dean and Jett [71]. Few algorithms will handle every histogram, particularly if the data are noisy, the CV large, or the cell cycle severely distorted. The numbers generated should not be blindly accepted but instead used in conjunction with the original DNA histogram. Note also that the numbers produced by the computer program are only estimates.

The two most commonly used commercial DNA analysis software packages are ModFit (Verity Software) and Multicycle (Phoenix Flow Systems). Figure 5.4 shows a computer analysis of some DNA histograms produced with ModFit.

Some general guidelines are as follows:

1. Determine the cell ploidy and report the DNA index of all ploidy populations.
2. Report the CV of the main G0G1 peak. Generally, less than three is good and more than eight is poor.
3. When measuring the S-phase fraction (SPF) of a diploid tumor, make a statement as to whether the S phase was measured on the

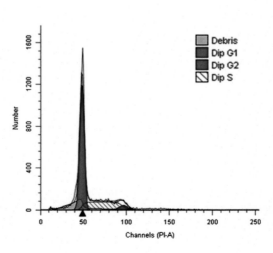

Fig. 5.4 Cell cycle analysis using ModFit software

File analyzed: Sample 1.fcs
Date analyzed: 31-May-2013
Model: 1Dn0n_DSD
Analysis type: Manual analysis

Ploidy Mode: First cycle is diploid

Diploid: 100.00%
  Dip G1: 65.99% at 48.41
  Dip G2: 4.85% at 96.83
  Dip S: 29.16% G2/G1: 2.00
  %CV: 5.42

Total S-Phase: 29.16%
Total B.A.D.: 8.08% no aggs

Debris: 17.23%
Aggregates: 0.00%
Modeled events: 14616
All cycle events: 12098
Cycle events per channel: 245
RCS: 5.149

whole sample, including normal cells, or on the tumor cells alone, gated by tumor-specific antibody.

4. Add a brief comment if necessary to cover any other information that may be helpful to someone looking at the result (e.g., inadequate number of cells, high debris levels, high CV, % background, aggregates, and debris).

Generally, a result should be rejected if any of the following apply:

1. CV of the G0G1 peak is greater than 8 %.
2. Sample contains fewer than 10,000–20,000 nuclei.
3. Data contain more than 30 % debris.
4. Flow rate was too high, as indicated by a broad CV or curved populations on two-parameter plots.
5. G0G1 peak is not in channel 200 of 1024 or 100 of 512 (i.e., on a suitable scale in a known channel).
6. Fewer than 200 cells in S phase (if SPF is to be reported).
7. G0G1 to G2M ratio is not between 1.95 and 2.05.

Instrument Setup for Cell Cycle Analyses

The instrument settings are also critical to obtaining a good histogram. Instrument setup varies with manufacturer. However, some general principles to observe are as follows:

1. Select the LIN channel that is most appropriate for the DNA probe.
2. Set the trigger on the channel detecting the DNA probe, as light scatter parameters are not usually of much use for triggering in the case of DNA.
3. Select parameters to enable doublet discrimination.
4. Set a gate to exclude doublets and apply it to the histogram that will display the DNA

profile. Displaying an ungated plot of the same may data may also be useful.

5. Make sure the sheath tank is full, as it may help with stability.
6. Make sure the cytometer is clean. Stream disruption will increase the CV.
7. Set a low flow rate and dilute cells to a concentration that is appropriate for the DNA probe solution.
8. Make sure the instrument has been optimized by running routine calibration particles.

Flow Cytometric Cell Sorting

Flow sorting is a process that allows the physical separation of a cell or particle of interest from a heterogeneous population. Sorting is an elegant use of flow cytometric technology that is attracting new attention from the diverse fields of biology and industry.

This technology provides the powerful yet unique ability to rapidly isolate pure populations of cells or particles with a desired set of biological characteristics. These populations are then available for morphological or genetic examination as well as functional assays and therapeutics. The main applications of flow sorting are as follows:

1. Single-cell cloning of hybridoma cells for the production of monoclonal antibodies
2. Isolating and purifying stem and/or progenitor cells
3. Sorting transfected cells with an expression marker, such as green fluorescence protein
4. Multiparameter isolation of cells from mixed populations
5. Sorting spermatozoa utilizing the difference in DNA content between those bearing the X and Y chromosomes
6. Single-cell sorting for clonogenic assays

In this context, although flow sorters are primarily used to sort mammalian cells, it is more accurate to refer to particle sorting given that flow sorters have also been used to sort yeast

[72], bacteria [73], and phytoplankton [74]. Flow sorting is the only practical way of isolating large numbers of specific chromosomes from humans, other primates [75], or plant species [76], and flow sorters proved invaluable during the human genome sequencing project [75] and more recently in the production of chromosome paints [76]. In addition, as the newer scientific fields of genomics and proteomics have evolved, flow sorting has become important in, for example, sorting large numbers of specific subsets of cells for microarray analysis [77]. At the other end of the scale, single particles may also be sorted into individual wells of a plate for cloning [78] or for PCR analysis [79]. Therefore, the applications of flow sorting are range widely, and a flow sorter, or access to one, is an invaluable resource.

Two methods exist for sorting particles by flow cytometry: electrostatic and mechanical. For the electrostatic method, the particles are passed in a stream of fluid out through a narrow orifice, at which point they pass through a laser beam and are analyzed in the same way as in a standard flow cytometer. A vibration is passed to the sample stream, which causes it to break into droplets at a stable break-off point. If a particle of interest passes through the laser beam, it is identified; when it reaches the droplet of the break-off point, an electric charge (positive or negative) is applied to the stream. As the droplet leaves the stream, it passes through deflection plates carrying a high voltage, and the droplet will be attracted to one of these plates, depending on the charge it was given. Uncharged droplets pass through un-deflected, and deflected droplets are collected in tubes. Thus, two or more different populations of particles can be sorted from the one sample. Most of the high-speed cell sorters use the electrostatic deflection of droplets method.

With the mechanical method, particles of interest are diverted within the flow cell, either by moving a "catcher" tube into the stream or by deflecting them with an acoustic pulse into a fixed tube. Briefly, the catcher tube is located in the upper portion of the flow cell and moves into the stream to collect the particles. When particles pass through the laser beam, the system determines whether each cell belongs to the selected population defined by boundaries in the cytogram. If the particle is identified as being of interest, it is captured by the catcher tube and collected into a tube or into a concentration module; otherwise it is dispatched to the waste tank.

The main drawback of mechanical sorting is the possibility to sort only one population of cells at a slow speed. Nevertheless, no aerosol is involved, which means it is safe to sort samples that have been treated with toxic substances such as radioactive compounds.

The advantage of electrostatic sorting is the ability to sort two subpopulations of cells at a high speed. However, it generates aerosols, so it is not appropriate to sort samples that have been treated with toxic substances. The high pressure generated in electrostatic sorting can also damage the sorted cells.

For precise sorting it is very important to adjust several parameters, including the following:

- The nozzle vibration conditioned by the drop drive frequency (ddf; the number of drops formed per second) and its amplitude level, the particle rate, i.e., the speed, which influences the distance between each cell.
- The dead time: time taken by the instrument to measure a particle's signal and reset to measure the next particle (i.e., time necessary to analyze one particle).
- The drop delay: distance between the laser beam interception of the cell and the break-off point, the point where the stream beaks into droplets.

In addition, other important parameters used to describe the success of cell sorting are yield, recovery, and purity. Yield is the proportion of sorted particles of interest compared with the total number of particles of interest that could have been recovered under ideal conditions. Recovery is the proportion of sorted particles of interest compared with the total number of particles of interest satisfying the sort decision.

Purity is the proportion of sorted particles of interest compared with the total number of particles in the sorted material. Purity can be, and often is, very high (>98 %), but a simple approach to how the material is re-analyzed can often lead to apparently lower purities than are actually achieved.

Sample Preparation for Cell Sorting and Setup

Sample preparation prior to sorting is important; in fact, successful sorting depends almost entirely on the state of the input sample. It is a prerequisite for flow cytometry that cells or particles be in a monodispersed suspension. This is relatively easy when the cells used are in a natural suspension (e.g., blood cells or suspension-cultured cells) but more problematic when using cells from adherent cultures or from solid tissue. However, several methods for preparing samples for flow sorting are well established. The main steps for preparing samples from suspension cells are as follows:

1. Take cells directly from the flask into 50-ml conical tubes and centrifuge at 800 g for 6 min.
2. Discard the supernatant and re-suspend in medium (cell culture medium or PBS with 1 % bovine serum albumin).
3. Centrifuge again at 800 g and discard supernatant. Count cells and re-suspend at an appropriate concentration, which will vary with sorter used. The final suspension medium will depend on the cell types to be sorted. In general, a low protein concentration is recommended because this will lead to less cell clumping.

In addition, samples from adherent cells should be prepared as follows:

1. Harvest cells using trypsin or versene. Transfer cells to 50-ml conical tubes and centrifuge at 400 g for 5 min.
2. Discard the supernatant and re-suspend in medium (cell culture medium or PBS with 1 % bovine serum albumin).

3. Centrifuge again at 800 g and discard supernatant. Re-suspend the cells in a small volume of medium and aspirate up and down through a pipette several times to help disaggregate clumps. Count cells and re-suspend at an appropriate concentration. In practice, adherent cells tend to be larger, and a lower concentration is recommended. It is always better to keep the concentration high prior to sorting and dilute to an appropriate concentration immediately prior to a sort.

Finally, the main steps for preparing cells from solid tissue are as follows:

1. Place tissue in a sterile Petri dish. Tease tissue apart using a needle and scalpel or alternatively use an automated system such as a MediMachine (Consults, Italy) [80]. In addition, enzymatic disaggregation (e.g., collagenase or dispase) may also help free single cells.
2. Decant cells into a 50-ml conical tube and centrifuge at 800 g for 6 min.
3. Discard the supernatant and re-suspend in medium (cell culture medium or PBS with 1 % bovine serum albumin).
4. Centrifuge again at 800 g and discard supernatant. Re-suspend the cells in a small volume of medium and count cells as above.

All preparations may be filtered through sterile nylon mesh prior to sorting; a range of pore sizes from 20 to 70 μm will be suitable for most cell types encountered.

Another central concern that must be considered has to do with procedures for sorting setup. It is important to ensure all fluidics lines are cleaned and/or replaced regularly. If a sort is aseptic (i.e., one in which cells will be required to be re-cultured or transplanted), a sterilization procedure will be needed. In general, this involves running 70 % ethanol through all fluidics lines for 30–60 min before flushing with distilled water (30 min) and finally sterile sheath fluid (at least 30 min before commencing a sort). All areas where the cells can potentially be in contact with the atmosphere (i.e., the sample line and sort chamber) should also be cleaned with ethanol prior to a sort. To check the sterility of a flow sorter, it is useful to periodically remove fluid from key locations (sheath tank, nozzle, and sample line) and put this into culture in an appropriate medium; cultures should remain sterile for at least 7 days.

The next consideration is nozzle size. The cell type will influence the size of orifice used. A general rule of thumb is that for blockage-free sorting and coherent side streams, a cell should be no more than one-fifth the diameter of the nozzle. In practice, this means that small round cells such as lymphocytes would require a 70-μm nozzle, whereas many cultured adherent cell lines and primary cells such as keratinocytes would require a 100-μm nozzle.

The third consideration is the laser alignment. The laser or lasers must hit the stream in parallel and the beams must be focused correctly.

Alignment may be checked using fluorescent beads that are excited by a particular wavelength of light and have a broad emission spectrum; it is also important to monitor the sensitivity of the sorter using multipeak beads with a variety of fluorescence intensities. The number of lasers used and the fluorochromes to be detected will also vary and need to be determined before the flow sorter is prepared. Once aligned, the frequency and amplitude of the drop must be found to obtain a stable break-off point. The latter will be found at several harmonic resonance frequencies, and the ability to find the most stable of these comes with operator experience. Many modern sorters can automatically detect movement of the break-off point and change the amplitude accordingly. The principles of sorting are relatively straightforward, but successful sorting is very much a result of experience; a basic grounding in and understanding of lasers, fluidics, computing, and biology are essential if a flow sorter is to be used to its full potential.

Data Analyses

Numerous software options are available for the analysis of flow cytometric data. One possibility involves histograms that show fluorescence patterns of a population for a single parameter, as represented in Fig. 5.5.

The histogram shows the FITC fluorescence pattern for collagen II of human primary chondrocytes. First, at the moment of analysis, the researcher must always perform a dot plot for physical parameters, defining a gate that delimits the cell population of interest. The gate is important because it excludes events such as cell debris that can affect the analysis.

The operator can then undertake different analyses independent of software. In this case, as reported in Table 5.4, the percentage of cells, the percentage of gated cells, and the geometric mean were obtained.

For many applications, such as phenotypic characterization, data collection on a logarithmic scale is preferred to a linear scale. An overlay constitutes a specialized type of histogram that permits the simultaneous display of parameter

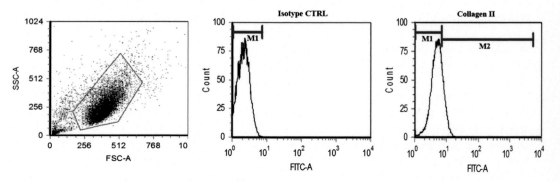

Fig. 5.5 Dot plot for physical parameters and histograms for isotype control and collagen II

Table 5.4 Analyses of cells expressing collagen II

Histogram#	Filename	Parameter	Marker	#Events	% of all cells	% of gated cells	Geometric mean
1	chondro-41	FITC-A	M1	7840	66.7	79.71	4.4
1	chondro-41	FITC-A	M2	2148	18.27	21.84	8.9

data from multiple samples, as reported in Fig. 5.6.

With this approach, individual samples can be compared based on a specific fluorescent or light scatter parameter, or control data can be overlayed against test samples to distinguish experimental significance. This type of analysis is performed to screen for the expression of specific proteins from reporter gene constructs, identifying cell lines with anomalous gene expression patterns, or monitoring gene expression of a population in response to external factors such as biologically significant compounds.

Alternate methods of data display are available for two-parameter plots. One option is contouring, which displays the data as a series of lines, similar to that observed with topographical maps. The contour patterns correlate to the distribution and density levels of cells or particles within the plot and can be used to aid in data analysis or to delineate populations of interest.

Various statistics are available for assessing the data within histograms and dot plots. Common statistics include total counts, population percentages, mean, median, CV, and SD. For example, total counts and percentages for specific cell populations can often be used in the clinical diagnosis of disease. In the case of HIV-infected patients, assessment of the T cells expressing the cell-surface proteins CD4 and CD8 can be used to determine a patient's immunological status. The CV statistic is traditionally used in conjunction with beads for calibration and daily quality control of the instrument, while the mean can be used to quantify the fluorescent intensity of a cell using standard calibration units or molecules of equivalent soluble fluorochrome (MESF). Regions can be created within histograms and dot plots to generate

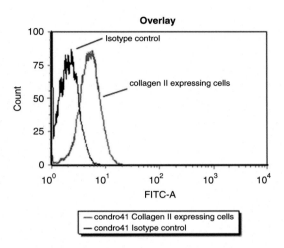

Fig. 5.6 Overlay. Primary chondrocytes were stained and analyzed using fluorescein isothiocyanate (FITC)-conjugated anti-collagen II antibody

statistics on subpopulations. In the case of disease diagnosis, clinicians often rely on the statistics from various lymphocyte subsets to characterize and treat many types of leukemia and lymphoma. Study of these disorders is typically based on identifying those cells containing certain expression patterns of cell-surface proteins. Factors such as total cell count, population percentages, "brightness" or fluorescent differences between populations, or statistical ratios between populations can then be used to analyze and quantitatively assess the data.

Regions can also be used for the creation and application of gates. Gates may involve one or more regions and are used primarily to minimize or eliminate extraneous events within an analysis plot or to isolate specific cells and particles of interest. Some software programs also provide the ability to assign colors to those events that fall within a particular region or gate, thus enabling easy identification of those cells within other histograms or dot plots.

Compensation

Another important consideration when conducting multicolor experiments is the possibility of fluorescence interference created by dyes or fluorochromes that possess close or overlapping emission spectra. In flow cytometry, this process is known as compensation. Compensation refers to specific software or hardware manipulations that mathematically remove fluorescence overlap to simplify multicolor data interpretation and distinguish populations on a dual-parameter histogram.

One benefit of this process is that it ultimately enables researchers to better delineate populations based on the expression or non-expression of specific cellular components, such as cell-surface antigens. Compensation currently represents one of the foremost obstacles to conducting multiparameter experiments in flow cytometry. Therefore, the experience of operator is also very important.

Conclusions

In summary, flow cytometry is an interesting tool for characterization of cells, ploidy level of tissues, nuclear DNA content, division frequency (through the detailed analysis of cell cycles), and phenotypic characterization. Flow cytometers are distinguished by their capacity to collect and process large amounts of data expeditiously. With a system to detect, view, and analyze the expression patterns of multiple proteins involved in complex biological processes such as apoptosis, oncogenesis, or cell division, investigators are better able to understand the possible combinatorial roles that specific proteins play in these processes and to provide data for diagnosis and ongoing patient treatment.

The advantages of flow cytometry, including data storage and analysis, ensure the prominence of this science in the continued study and understanding of complex cellular processes.

References

1. Ashcroft RG, Lopez PA. Commercial high speed machines open new opportunities in high throughput flow cytometry (HTFC). J Immunol Methods. 2000;243:13–24.
2. Hawley TS, Telford WG, Ramezani A, Hawley RG. Four-color flow cytometric detection of retrovirally expressed red, yellow, green, and cyan fluorescent proteins. Biotechniques. 2001;30:1028–34.
3. Rosen ED, Husi C, Wang X, Sakai S, et al. C/EBPα induces adipogenesis through PPAR: a unified pathway. Genes Dev. 2002;16:22.
4. Feldhaus M, Siegel R. Flow cytometric screening of yeast surface display libraries. Methods Mol Biol. 2004;263:311–32.
5. Moldavan A. Photo-electric technique for the counting of microscopical cells. Science. 1934;80:188–9.
6. Gucker Jr FT, O'Konski CT, Pickard HB, Pitts Jr JN. A photoelectronic counter for colloidal particles. J Am Chem Soc. 1947;69:2422–31.
7. Cornwall JB, Davison RM. Rapid counter for small particles in suspension. J Sci Instrum. 1950;37:414–6.
8. Coulter WH. High speed automatic blood cell counter and analyzer. Proc Natl Electron Conf. 1956;12:1034–40.
9. Bierne T, Hutcheon JM. A photoelectric particle counter for use in the sieve range. J Sci Instrum. 1957;34:196–200.
10. Kamentsky LA, Melamed MR. Spectrophotometer: new instrument for ultrarapid cell analysis. Science. 1965;150:630–1.
11. Kamentsky LA, Melamed MR. Spectrophotometric cell sorter. Science. 1967;156:1364–5.
12. Fulwyler MJ. Electronic separation of biological cells by volume. Science. 1965;150:910–1.
13. Dittrich W, Göhde W. Impulsfluorometrie dei einzelzellen in suspensionen. Z Naturforsch. 1969;24b:360–1.
14. Van Dilla MA, Trujillo TT, Mullaney PF, Coulter JR. Cell microfluorimetry: a method for rapid fluorescence measurement. Science. 1969;163:1213–4.
15. Hulett HR, Bonner WA, Barrett J, Herzenberg LA. Cell sorting: automated separation of mammalian cells as a function of intracellular fluorescence. Science. 1969;166:747–9.
16. Shapiro HM. Practical flow cytometry. 4th ed. New York: Wiley-Liss; 2003.
17. Melamed MR, Mullaney PF, Shapiro HM. An historical review of the development of flow cytometers and sorters. In: Melamed MR, Lindmo T, Mendelsohn ML, editors. Flow cytometry and sorting. 2nd ed. New York: Wiley-Liss; 1990. p. 1–8.
18. Melamed MR. A brief history of flow cytometry and sorting. Methods Cell Biol. 2001;63:3–16.

19. Romanowsky D. Zur Frage der Parasitologie und Therapie der Malaria. St Petersburg Med Wochenschr. 1891;16:297–302, 307–15.
20. Horobin RW, Walter KJ. Understanding Romanowsky staining. I: The Romanowsky-Giemsa effect in blood smears. Histochemistry. 1987;86:331–6.
21. Ehrlich P. Methodologische Beiträge zur Physiologie und Pathologie der verschiedenen Formen der Leukocyten. Z Klin Med. 1880;1:553–60.
22. Dittrich W, Göhde W. Impulse fluorometry of single cells in suspension. Z Naturforsch B. 1969;24:360–1.
23. Crissman HA, Steinkamp JA. Rapid, simultaneous measurement of DNA, protein, and cell volume in single cells from large mammalian cell populations. J Cell Biol. 1973;59:766–71.
24. Crissman HA, Tobey RA. Cell-cycle analysis in 20 minutes. Science. 1974;184:1297–8.
25. Latt SA, Stetten G. Spectral studies on 33258 Hoechst and related bisbenzimidazole dyes useful for fluorescent detection of deoxyribonucleic acid synthesis. J Histochem Cytochem. 1976;24:24–33.
26. Stöhr M, Eipel H, Goerttler K, Vogt-Schaden M. Extended application of flow microfluorometry by means of dual laser excitation. Histochemistry. 1977;51:305–13.
27. Coons AH, Creech HJ, Jones RN, Berliner E. Demonstration of pneumococcal antigen in tissues by use of fluorescent antibody. J Immunol. 1942;45:159–70.
28. Kano K, Loza U, Gerbasi JR, Milgrom F. Studies on heterophile antibodies in transplantation sera. Transplantation. 1975;19:20–6.
29. http://whcf.org/WHCF WallaceHCoulter.htm
30. Ingram M, Preston Jr K. Automatic analysis of blood cells. Sci Am. 1970;223:72–82.
31. Prewitt JMS, Mendelsohn ML. The analysis of cell images. Ann N Y Acad Sci. 1966;128:1035–53.
32. Fulwyler MJ. An electronic particle separator with potential biological application. Los Alamos Scientific Laboratory Annual Report of the Biological and Medical Research Group (H–4) of the Health Division, July 1964–June 1965, Written July 1965.
33. Mullaney PF, Dean PN. Cell sizing: a small-angle light-scattering method for sizing particles of low relative refractive index. Appl Opt. 1969;8:2361–2.
34. "The History of the Cell Sorter Interviews". Record Unit 9554. Smithsonian Institution Archives. Retrieved 9 Mar 2012.
35. Stubblefield E, Cram S, Deaven L. Flow microfluorometric analysis of isolated Chinese hamster chromosomes. Exp Cell Res. 1975;94:464–8.
36. van den Engh GJ, Trask BJ, Gray JW, Langlois RG, et al. Preparation and bivariate analysis of suspensions of human chromosomes. Cytometry. 1985;6:92–100.
37. Lloyd D. Flow cytometry in microbiology. London: Springer; 1993.
38. Shapiro HM. Microbial analysis at the single-cell level: tasks and techniques. J Microbiol Methods. 2000;42:3–16.
39. Fugger EF, Black SH, Keyvanfar K, Schulman JD. Births of normal daughters after MicroSort sperm separation and intrauterine insemination, in-vitro fertilization, or intracytoplasmic sperm injection. Hum Reprod. 1998;13:2367–70.
40. Gledhill BL, Evenson DP, Pinkel D. Flow cytometry and sorting of sperm and male germ cells. In: Melamed MR, Lindmo T, Mendelsohn ML, editors. Flow cytometry and sorting. 2nd ed. New York: Wiley-Liss; 1990. p. 531–51.
41. Reckerman M, Collin F. Aquatic flow cytometry: achievements and prospects. Science. 2000;64:235–46.
42. Marie D, Brussard CPD, Thyrhaug R, Bratbak G, et al. Enumeration of marine viruses in culture and natural samples by flow cytometry. Appl Environ Microbiol. 1999;59:905–11.
43. Hedley DW. Flow cytometry using paraffin-embedded tissue: five years on. Cytometry. 1989;10:229–41.
44. Gray JW, Cram LS. Flow karyotyping and chromosome sorting. In: Melamed MR, Lindmo T, Mendelsohn ML, editors. Flow cytometry and sorting. 2nd ed. New York: Wiley-Liss; 1990.
45. Habbersett RC, Jett JH, Keller RA. Single DNA fragment detection by flow cytometry. In: Durack G, Robinson JP, editors. Emerging tools for single-cell analysis. New York: Wiley-Liss; 2000. p. 115–38.
46. Carson RT, Vignali DAA. Simultaneous quantitation of 15 cytokines using a multiplexed flow cytometric assay. J Immunol Methods. 1999;227:41–52.
47. Brown M, Wittwer C. Flow cytometry: principles and clinical applications in hematology. Clin Chem. 2000;46:1221–9.
48. Dal Bó S, Pezzi A, Amorin B, Valim V, et al. Detection of minimal residual disease by flow cytometry for patients with multiple myeloma submitted to autologous hematopoietic stem cell transplantation. ISRN Hematol. 2013;2013:847672. doi:10.1155/2013/847672.
49. Harrington AM, Olteanu H, Kroft SH. A dissection of the CD45/side scatter "blast gate". Am J Clin Pathol. 2012;137:800–4.
50. Stacchini A, Demurtas A, Godio L, Martini G, et al. Flow cytometry in the bone marrow staging of mature B-cell neoplasms. Cytometry B Clin Cytom. 2003;54:10–8.
51. Ruiz-Arguelles A, Duque RE, Orfao A. Report on the first Latin American Consensus Conference for Flow Cytometric Immunophenotyping of Leukemia. Cytometry. 1998;34:39–42.
52. Di Giuseppe JA, Borowitz MJ. Clinical utility of flow cytometry in the chronic lymphoid leukemias. Semin Oncol. 1998;25:6–10.

53. Davis BH, Foucar K, Szczarkowski W, Ball E, et al. U.S.-Canadian Consensus recommendations on the immunophenotypic analysis of hematologic neoplasia by flow cytometry: medical indications. Cytometry. 1997;30:249–63.

54. Grier DD, Al-Quran SZ, Cardona DM, Li Y, et al. Flow cytometric analysis of immunoglobulin heavy chain expression in B-cell lymphoma and reactive lymphoid hyperplasia. Int J Clin Exp Pathol. 2012;5:110–8.

55. Joensuu H, Klemi PJ. DNA aneuploidy in adenomas of endocrine organs. Am J Pathol. 1988;132:145–51.

56. Joensuu H, Klemi P, Eerola E. DNA aneuploidy in follicular adenomas of the thyroid gland. Am J Pathol. 1986;124:373–6.

57. Hedley DW, Shankey TV, Wheeless LL. DNA cytometry consensus conference. Cytometry. 1993;14:471.

58. Friedlander ML, Hedley DW, Taylor IW. Clinical and biological significance of aneuploidy in human tumours. J Clin Pathol. 1984;37:961–74.

59. Duque RE, Andreeff M, Braylan RC, Diamond LW, et al. Consensus review of the clinical utility of DNA flow cytometry in neoplastic hematopathology. Cytometry. 1993;14:492–6.

60. Albro J, Bauer KD, Hitchcock CL, Wittwer CT. Improved DNA content histograms from formalin-fixed, paraffin-embedded liver tissue by proteinase K digestion. Cytometry. 1993;14:673–8.

61. Look AT, Roberson PK, Williams DL, Rivera G, et al. Prognostic importance of blast cell DNA content in childhood acute lymphoblastic leukemia. Blood. 1985;65:1079–86.

62. Dressler LG, Bartow SA. DNA flow cytometry in solid tumors: practical aspects and clinical applications. Semin Diagn Pathol. 1989;6:55–82.

63. Gunawan B, Fuzesi L, Granzen B, Keller U, et al. Clinical aspects of alveolar rhabdomyosarcoma with translocation t(1;13)(p36;q14) and hypotetraploidy. Pathol Oncol Res. 1999;5:211–3.

64. Gollin SM, Janecka IP. Cytogenetics of cranial base tumors. J Neurooncol. 1994;20:241–54.

65. Ormerod MG. Flow cytometry: a practical approach. 3rd ed. Oxford: IRL Press at Oxford University Press; 2000. p. 235–46.

66. Darzynkiewicz Z, Paul Robinson J, Crissman HA. Methods in cell biology: flow cytometry vol 42, Part B, 2nd ed., 1994. 15. Practical flow cytometry, 3rd ed., Shapiro, 1994.

67. Vindeløv LL, Christensen IJ, Nissen NI. A detergent-trypsin method for the preparation of nuclei for flow cytometric DNA analysis. Cytometry. 1983;3:323–6.

68. Hedley DW, Friedlander ML, Taylor IW, Rugg CA, et al. Method for analysis of cellular DNA content of paraffin embedded pathological material using flow cytometry. J Histochem Cytochem. 1983;31:1333–3335.

69. Leers MP, Schutte B, Theunissen PH, Ramaekers FC, et al. Heat pretreatment increases resolution in DNA flow cytometry of paraffin-embedded tumor tissue. Cytometry. 1999;35:260–6.

70. Rabinovitch PS. DNA content histogram and cell-cycle analysis. Methods Cell Biol. 1994;41:263–96.

71. Dean PN, Jett JH. Mathematical analysis of DNA distributions derived from flow microfluorometry. J Cell Biol. 1974;60:523–6.

72. Deere D, Shen J, Vesey G, Bell P, et al. Flow cytometry and cell sorting for yeast viability assessment and cell selection. Yeast. 1998;14:147–60.

73. Sekar R, Fuchs BM, Amann R, Pernthaler J. Flow sorting of marine bacterioplankton after fluorescence in situ hybridization. Appl Environ Microbiol. 2004;70:6210–9.

74. Jochem FJ. Short-term physiologic effects of mechanical flow sorting and the Becton-Dickinson cell concentrator in cultures of the marine phytoflagellata Emiliania huxleyi and Micromonas pusilla. Cytometry. 2005;65:77–83.

75. Ferguson-Smith MA, Yang F, Rens W, O'Brien PC. The impact of chromosome sorting and painting on the comparative analysis of primate genomes. Cytogenet Genome Res. 2005;108:112–21.

76. Dolezel J, Kubalakova M, Bartos J, Macas J. Flow cytogenetics and plant genome mapping. Chromosome Res. 2004;12:77–91.

77. Szaniszlo P, Wang N, Sinha M, et al. Getting the right cells to the array: gene expression microarray analysis of cell mixtures and sorted cells. Cytometry. 2004;59:191–202.

78. Battye FL, Light A, Tarlinton DM. Single cell sorting and cloning. J Immunol Methods. 2000;243:25–32.

79. Williams C, Davies D, Williamson R. Segregation of F508 and normal CFTR alleles in human sperm. Hum Mol Genet. 1993;2:445–8.

80. Molnar B, Bocsi J, Karman J, et al. Immediate DNA ploidy analysis of gastrointestinal biopsies taken by endoscopy using a mechanical dissociation device. Anticancer Res. 2003;23:655–60.

Advanced Imaging Techniques

6

C. Cavaliere, M. Aiello, E. Torino, V. Mollo, L. Marcello,
D. De Luca, N. Pignatelli di Spinazzola, V. Parlato,
and P.A. Netti

Microscopy in Cells, Tissues, and Organs: Main Strategies in Sample Preparation and Observation

Introduction

An understanding of normal cell activity is crucial to allow us to observe variations throughout the cell cycle as well as responses to altered circumstances such as stress and disease. Electron microscopy (EM) has profoundly influenced our understanding of tissue organization and especially cells by allowing us to visualize molecules and even atoms.

Since 1930, the much shorter wavelength of the electron began to open the submicroscopic world to our view. EM added another thousand-fold increase in magnification over light microscopy, accompanied by a parallel increase in resolution capability at the Angstrom level. This enabled scientists to visualize viruses, DNA, and many other smaller organelles or substructured biological materials.

Many of the biologists who pioneered biological EM are still alive; it was only in 1974 that George Palade was awarded the Nobel Prize in Medicine for his accomplishments in cell biology using EM.

Numerous methodologies for tissue preparation, sectioning, and analysis were later developed to use EM for specific problems. These techniques were at first in the hands of only a few investigators and varied greatly between laboratories. Recently, most of these techniques have been standardized and are now freely available to everyone.

It is important to note that the nature of EM does not allow the imaging of live cells or observations of dynamic events within the cell; instead, EM provides a snapshot of the events occurring at the initial EM observation. To select the point of initial observation, EM preparation must be run in parallel with live cell imaging, and

C. Cavaliere (✉) • M. Aiello
NAPLab - IRCCS SDN, Naples, Italy
e-mail: ccavaliere@sdn-napoli.it

E. Torino • V. Mollo
Center for Advanced Biomaterials for Health Care
(CABHC), Istituto Italiano di Tecnologia, Naples, Italy

L. Marcello
Institute of Human Anatomy, Seconda Università degli
Studi di Napoli, Naples, Italy

D. De Luca
U.O. Fisica Sanitaria - P.O. "V. Faze", Lecce, Italy

N. Pignatelli di Spinazzola • V. Parlato
Department of Radiological Sciences, Seconda
Università degli Studi di Napoli, Naples, Italy

P.A. Netti
Center for Advanced Biomaterials for Health Care
CABHC - Istituto Italiano di Tecnologia, Naples, Italy

CRIB – Centro di Ricerca Interdipartimentale sui
Biomateriali – Università Federico II di Napoli, Naples,
Italy

© Springer Science+Business Media New York 2016
F.M. Sacerdoti et al. (eds.), *Advanced Imaging Techniques in Clinical Pathology*,
Current Clinical Pathology, DOI 10.1007/978-1-4939-3469-0_6

the sample must be preserved before the EM observations. Traditional techniques for EM sample preparation involve chemical fixation and resin infiltration, with the disadvantage that the process is slow and invasive. It therefore has great potential to induce changes and include artifacts.

Recent advances in scanning electron microscopy (SEM) and transmission electron microscopy (TEM), combining freezing and embedding techniques, have provided excellent results in terms of "instant" stabilization of the biological matrix and sufficient contrast of subcellular elements; however, a spectrum of approaches must be considered, keeping the required end point in mind. The type of EM used should also be considered when applying EM to investigations of subcellular structure. Very little of the work published on cellular EM mentions SEM and the advantages of TEM. Since the advent of field emission SEM (FE-SEM), which provides SEM with the same resolution as TEM for biological material, recent results have shown the combined FE-SEM/TEM approach can provide multi-scale observations of cellular substructures. In particular, while TEM provides localized information about a specific section of cells, organs, or tissues, FE-SEM provides information about the surfaces and interfaces at which many phenomena occur. This multi-scale approach has been widely used in the newly developed field of nanotechnologies in biology. In particular, customized nanoparticles have been developed to deliver drugs directly to diseased cells or to improve the performance of contrast agents or radiotracers. Multi-scale observations are necessary to fully understand the nano–bio interfaces and all the interactions that occur between nanoparticles and biological counterparts such as DNA/RNA (a few Angstroms to a few nanometers), proteins (up to tens of nanometers), lipid cellular membrane (up to hundreds of nanometers), and so on.

Scope

This chapter provides an overview of recent advances in EM and sample preparation techniques for cells, tissues, and organs. We first provide a general introduction about the importance of EM when applied to biological samples. We then describe the basic principles of cryo-EM and tomographic data acquisition and image processing, discussing their relative advantages and disadvantages. We further discuss how recent advances in instrumentation and methodology have led electron tomography (ET) to become the highest-resolution three-dimensional (3D) imaging technique for unique objects such as cells (Figs. 6.1 and 6.2).

Technique Description

Basic Principles and Advances in EM Observations for Tissues and Organs: Probe X-Ray Analysis, SEM, and TEM

Since the invention of EM nearly 80 years ago, researchers have been able to gain deep insights into biological structures. We start by discussing electron probe X-ray microanalysis, SEM, and TEM, and their applications, strategy, and advantages in anatomical pathology.

X-ray analysis has been most widely used for the study of biological specimens, as it can identify, localize, and quantify elements at both the whole-cell and the intracellular level. In addition to the use of SEM and TEM to analyze single and whole cells, it is a simple and rapid method of studying changes in ion transport as well as ionic content in intracellular compartments, such as mitochondria and lysosomes.

Among the element detection methods using EM, energy X-ray dispersive spectroscopy (EDS), also called electron probe X-ray microanalysis (EPXMA), is a powerful technique. In fact, at low resolution, EDS provides information about a large number of individual cells, overcoming the limits of common bulk chemical techniques such as atomic adsorption spectroscopy and fluorescent imaging at the light microscopy level. At high resolution, it is one of very few techniques that can provide information about single elements contained, for example, in the organelles. However, the technique is not suitable for the detection of

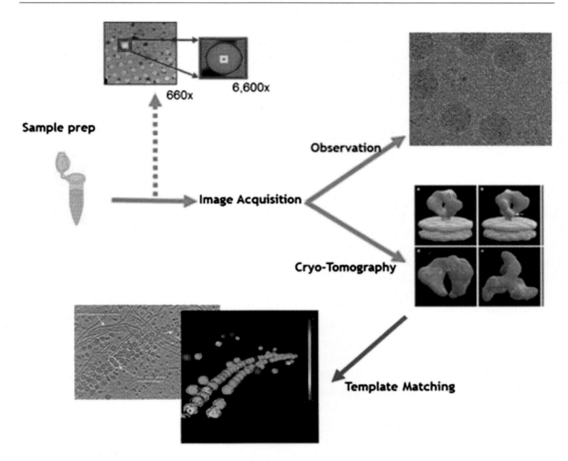

Fig. 6.1 Workflow of electron microscopy and 3D reconstruction

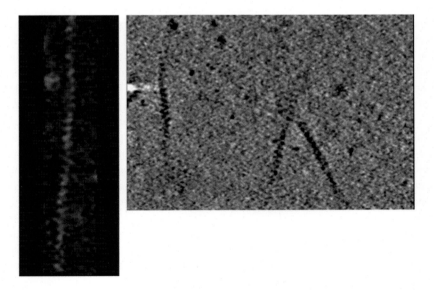

Fig. 6.2 Electron microscopy examples. (**a**) Surface rendering on reconstructed actin filament; (**b**) single z-slice taken from the reconstruction—Courtesy of FEI

elements present in very low concentrations (traces minus 100 ppm), and it cannot discriminate between bound and free forms. From this perspective, EDS has proved to be a powerful technique to match element composition and structural information. However, because of its need for high concentration, its application in the field of nanotechnology is limited, particularly in qualitative and quantitative approaches to nanoparticle detection within tissues, organs, and cells.

Given the above, there are some important considerations about using X-ray in conjunction with SEM and TEM. About 15 years after the development of the electron microscope by Knoll and Ruska in 1979, the first serious efforts were made to apply this technology to biological samples. EM has revolutionized our concept of cell structure and how cells interact. The basic principles have remained the same since its invention: the microscope column is under vacuum, allowing a beam of coherent electrons to be directed onto the specimen. Biological samples are mainly composed of light elements such as carbon, hydrogen, or oxygen with low electron densities and consequently low contrast in the electron beam. Moreover, in the TEM, the sample must be thin enough to allow the beam to penetrate into the sample; in the SEM, the sample must be conductive, to allow the beam to scan the surface of the sample.

When cells are analyzed using FE-SEM in combination with X-ray, the main problem affecting sensitivity is the over-penetration of the specimen by the electron beam. This causes excitation of the underlying substrate, altering the quantitative information. With combined X-ray and TEM, the acceleration voltage and the thickness of the section must be finely balanced. A high accelerating voltage decreases the scattering of electrons, improving the background. Some geometrical considerations between the detector, grid, and beam are required, and it is also very important that the analysis is conducted in the center of the grids as far as possible from the grid bars.

Some examples of SEM-EDS combinations in the study of apoptotic cell death are given by Arrebola et al. [1], and Zhang et al. [2] deal with the study of cardiac myocytes using EDS-TEM.

In conclusion, X-ray microanalysis is now being used in a variety of applications, with an emphasis on epithelial transport, the toxic effect of environmental pollutants, and in apoptotic and oncotic cell death mechanisms.

Sample Preservation with Freezing Techniques

Scientists have long studied the molecules that establish living cells in attempts to understand biological phenomena. The atomic resolution of the structure of DNA and proteins such as hemoglobin, myoglobin, and lysozyme were early triumphs in the emerging disciplines of molecular structural biology because these structures provided insights into molecular structures. Recent years have seen an explosion in the amount of information about the identity of molecular elements involved in cellular processes [3]. However, many assemblies are transient or not stable enough to be studied in vitro. Unfortunately, recreating in vivo conditions in vitro is often difficult. Therefore, EM can shorten the distance between ultrastructural compartmentalization and molecular structural analysis in cells.

To prepare a biological sample for EM, the first step is to arrest the biological activity of the specimen. Most of the time, in "conventional" protocols, aldehydes are used as a chemical fixative to cross-link the proteins. The reaction of aldehydes with lipids is limited and, even if the lipids are still in place after primary fixation, they might be extracted in the following steps. In "conventional" preparation, samples are treated by secondary fixation using osmium tetroxide (OsO_4), which not only reduces the extraction of lipids but also introduces contrast due to the deposition of the heavy metal onto the membrane [4, 5]. Tannic [6] and uranyl acetate [7, 8] are incorporated into the sample to improve membrane contrast. Unfortunately, in "conventional" protocols, samples are dehydrated using different solvents and infiltrated by a liquid resin, which is polymerized either by heat (for epoxy resin) [9] or by ultraviolet light for methacrylic resin. Once polymerized, the sample is cut into thin sections (50–200 nm) using an ultramicrotome and a diamond knife. Unfortunately, each of these preparation steps can insert artifacts that might damage some structure. In 1973, Tokuyasu [10] froze cell suspensions and tissue with a high-molarity sucrose solution as the cryoprotectant, where previously they have been fixed by aldehyde and embedded in gelatin. The sucrose prevents the formation of ice, and samples up to a volume of 1 mm^3 can be vitrified by plunging in liquid nitrogen [11]. Thin cryo-sections are cut from the frozen sample with a cryo-ultramicrotome (thickness 50–200 nm) and placed on to an EM grid with formvar film. Sections can be labeled with probes, antibodies, and in situ hybridization [12, 13]. In this procedure, freezing avoids resin embedding, but the fixative artifacts cannot be avoided.

With this success, freezing techniques were soon being used to arrest cellular and molecular processes. In fact, freezing is the initial step in an approach to EM preparation that is followed by dehydrating the sample at a low temperature (freeze-drying) and embedding it to allow sectioning at room temperature [14]. Artifacts associated with this method inspired the development of cryo-methods such as freeze fracture and superficial freeze-drying (etching) of samples at low temperatures [15, 16]. In SEM, samples are protected against structural collapse in the vacuum by full dehydration by critical point drying (CPD) after solvents and fixatives are used; however, dehydration may also induce shrinkage artifacts [17, 18]. Recent advances in EM sample preparation with improvements in the EM field have focused on imaging proteins, cells, and tissues in a state that is as close to their native state as possible. Nowadays, it seems as though the use of cryo-fixation is going to push electron microscopic resolution toward the imaging of macromolecular assemblies in intact cells and tissues. Cells contain not pure water, but ions, proteins, and sugar, which are soluble materials that interact with water molecules and change their behavior when frozen. Thus, the "water" in a sample must be vitrified to preserve

it in as lifelike a state as possible. When vitrification temperature is attained with rapid freezing, viscosity reaches a level that prevents movement, thus immobilizing all the molecules in a cell within milliseconds [19]. It has been shown that the formation of ice in cytoplasm induced phase segregation between water and solutes [20–22]. Furthermore, ice crystals cause holes in cellular membranes and destroy organelles [23]. To protect cell ultrastructure from deleterious ice crystal formation, biological samples are preincubated in a cryoprotectant solution such as dimethyl sulfoxide (DMSO), glycerol, or sucrose. However, these antifreeze agents cause different kinds of damage to the ultrastructure, such as shrinking, and specific responses to osmotic stress [23]. Plunge freezing is a simple method of obtaining the cooling rate required for vitrification. In this procedure, a very thin sample (<100 nm) is embedded in a thin layer of vitrified water and plunge frozen in liquid ethane, where the cooling rate reaches 108 K/s, before observation under a cryo-microscope. This method can be applied to single cells, bacteria, viruses, and isolated protein complexes [24]. It is not suitable for larger cells and tissue; in fact, these kinds of samples can be vitrified only a few micrometers into their surface [25–27]. Larger samples can be frozen by slam freezing, wherein the sample is propelled onto a metal surface that is cooled with helium or liquid nitrogen, so the sample surface is in direct contact with the cooled metal plate and cools quickly. It is suitable for samples with a maximum thickness of 20 µm [22]. The only practicable approach to vitrifying thicker samples is to reduce the cooling rate for vitrification by increasing pressure to 2100 bars during cooling [28]. This innovative approach is called high-pressure freezing (HPF). Before freezing, high pressure (2100 bars) is applied to the sample for a few milliseconds; at the same time the outer surface of the container that holds the samples is cooled with a jet of liquid nitrogen. Thus, the water in the sample becomes vitrified, but ice crystals do not have a chance to form. The advantages of HPF include the ability to freeze relatively large volumes (200 µm) without visible ice crystal damage; the procedure is generally reproducible; and it arrests and preserves molecules in a near-native state, making it an important tool for structural cell biology [29]. This approach is suitable for cell suspensions or small organisms such as *Caenorhabditis elegans* [30]; microbiopsies from various tissues [31, 32]; small organ pieces [33, 34], and vertebrate embryos. After sample collection, HPF is the second step in sample preparation; the next steps are required to process the vitreous sample into sections or replicas suitable for EM. There are four different follow-up procedures: (1) "freeze fracturing" [35] generates a replica of a fractured surface through the sample; (2) "freeze substitution" [36] and (3) "freeze-drying" produce a resin-embedded sample suitable for conventional sectioning with an ultramicrotome; and (4) "cryo-EM of vitreous sections" (CEMOVIS) is direct cryo-sectioning of a sample by a cryo-ultramicrotome, with the resulting frozen hydrated sections investigated on a cold stage in the electron microscope at $-170\ °C$ [37, 38].

Freeze fracturing provides superior structural preservation and is currently considered to be free of artifacts. This method enables investigation of the basic architecture of biological membranes and the mode of interaction between lipids and membrane proteins [39]. In combination with quick freezing, this method can deliver images of rapid biological processes such as synaptic vesicle release [40]. Freeze-drying is the en bloc freezing of a sample after cryo-fixation and embedding in resin; it enables the investigation of ion diffusion and is therefore used in secondary ion mass spectroscopy applications [41]. CEMOVIS [37] is the only TEM approach in which the real in situ structure is imaged directly. In this case, the micrograph is what remains from a sample after HPM, ultrathin sectioning, and exposure to an electron beam at $-170\ °C$. In contrast with freeze substitution, no chemical treatments are used that can precipitate or change the structure of the sample. With this method, it is possible to depict the structure of distinct macromolecular assemblies [42, 43]. Using CEMOVIS for recent studies of bacterial cytoskeletons, the organization of bacterial DNA, or the cell wall of mycobacterium has revealed new views on bacterial morphology and highlight the need for close to native state imaging [44–47].

Therefore, rapid freezing represents a good tool to immobilize tissue and cell samples. It also avoids ion and molecule leakage that occurs during conventional fixation at room temperature. Vitrification is the right way to go, followed by freeze substitution or frozen hydrated sectioning. In contrast to conventional preparation, freeze substitution offers improved morphological preservation. The stability of samples embedded in resin under the electron beam make this method an excellent choice for ET studies.

Visualizing Organ and Tissues Diseases with Cryo-Electron Microscopy

As mentioned, EM is a technique that is widely used in structural biology to solve the 3D structures of isolated macromolecular assemblies in situations that closely resemble their biological conditions [48]. The technique began with relatively simple "negatively stained" biological material deposited on electron microscope grids. Recently, ET has emerged as a novel approach to providing 3D information on cells and tissues at the molecular level. It is comparable to medical tomographic techniques such as positron emission tomography (PET)-magnetic resonance imaging (MRI) in that it provides a 3D view of an object with nanometric resolution. This characteristic allows researchers to visualize molecular assemblies, cytoskeleton elements, and organelles within cells, providing a 3D perspective of cellular organization in relation to disease-related morphological changes. The majority of cryo-ET studies performed in recent decades can be divided into four categories: (1) virus, (2) bacteria and eukaryotic cells, (3) organelles, and (4) macromolecular structures. In ET, tilted series of thick sections of plastic-embedded samples or thinner sections of vitrified samples are generally acquired with an electron microscope equipped with a eucentric tilt stage. The higher acceleration voltage (200–300 KV) enables the electron beam to penetrate the thick section. After acquisition, the single images of the tilt series are aligned, and algorithms are used to produce a 3D image. While a number of different algorithms exist, the commonly used is simultaneous iterative reconstruction technique (SIRT) [49]). Different software packages for alignment, reconstruction, and segmentation are available and are constantly evolving [50]. ET studies in HPF/freeze substitution-prepared samples are limited in resolution because of the presence of stain. It should be possible to increase resolution with unstained images from sections of vitrified samples. Unlike the ET of stained plastic sections, cryo-ET on vitreous sections (CETOVIS) of unstained cryosections has the potential to reach the resolution required for reliable interpretation at the molecular level with 3D imaging in the near to native state of the cellular structures. Combination with correlative light microscopy (LM) facilitates the search for features of interest, which otherwise can involve extensive scanning, as the field of view in EM is quite small compared with the size of a typical eukaryotic cell. Approaches combining LM with conventional EM preparation methods have clearly demonstrated the relevance of such techniques in cell biology [51]. Successful applications of correlative LM and cryo-ET on sparse cultures of immature neurons [52] and endothelial cells [53] have taken advantage of strong visual cues provided by large cellular features, which enabled the straightforward orientation of the sample

As discussed, the freezing approach avoids any chemical alteration or modification of the sample and preserves them in a condition very close to their native state, offering a higher resolution. It now seems that high-pressure freezing in combination with cryo-ET or cryo-EM will be the perfect method to enable visualization of the ultrastructure of living matter in a close to natural state. Cryo-ET stands out among imaging and structural biology methods. Cryo-tomograms of intact cells are a snapshot of the entire cellular proteome at a molecular resolution, which in principle will enable the mapping of spatial relationships between macromolecules and the cell [54]. Diverse identification strategies complementing cryo-ET with methods such as genetics and correlative fluorescence imaging are already being used, and new approaches are being explored. Immunolabeling with electron-dense markers suitable for living cells tends to be restricted to proteins with extracellular epitopes because the cell permeabilization methods used to label intracellular proteins induce significant structural changes [55]. Fluorescence microscopy has increased our understanding of cellular processes but has also left many questions unanswered regarding the molecular and supramolecular architecture of cellular complexes. The combination of correlative LM with cryo-ET enables imaging of the same features over multiple-length scales.

After a cryo-ET tilt series is recorded, the object is reconstructed from individual images by re-projection of all images from the aligned tilt series into a 3D volume. The most common techniques are back projection and algebraic reconstruction techniques (ART).

Some biological examples of cell observations with cryo-ET can be categorized by membrane structure such as mitochondria, Golgi apparatus, lysosomes, large protein structures, and virus structures. In conclusion, because the choice of specimen is not limited by its thickness in cryo-ET, the molecular basis of diseases is completely open for study.

Lesson Learned

We have reviewed how ET has begun to reveal the molecular organization of cells and how the existing and upcoming technologies promise even greater insights into structural cell biology. Advances in EM techniques offering resolution at the previously unattainable scale of a few nanometers are expected to provide novel insights into molecular structures. The role of X-ray microscopy and rapid freezing techniques combined (cryo-ET) is beginning to live up to expectations for their unique ability to provide 3D maps of the supramolecular organization in unperturbed cellular environments. Indeed, this technique helps to bridge the divide that existed, until now, between cellular and molecular structural studies. Furthermore, to extend cryo-ET to all kinds of cells and tissues, we must continue improving cryo-sectioning techniques to minimize disturbance from sectioning artifacts and to explore other methods of microdissection.

Two-Photon Microscopy

Introduction

Multiphoton fluorescence microscopy is a powerful tool that employs laser scanning microscopy and long-wavelength multiphoton fluorescence excitation to image high-resolution, volumetric scans of specimens labeled with specific fluorochromes [56, 57].

This methodology provides distinct advantages for 3D imaging, including the study of dynamic processes in living cells and especially within intact tissues such as brain slices, whole organs, and entire living animals [58, 59].

Although classical fluorescence microscopy can often achieve submicron resolution, the effective sensitivity, especially with thick specimens, is generally limited by background noise caused by scattering and autofluorescence of areas near the focal plane. Confocal microscopy can overcome some of the effects of scattering, since the detector pinhole rejects fluorescence from off-focus locations (Fig. 6.3). Nevertheless, scanning a single section excites, and thereby bleaches and damages, the entire specimen, significantly limiting the use of this technique in living tissues [60].

The natural evolution of confocal microscopy is represented by multiphoton imaging, where excitation is not focused on a single plane, as in the confocal setup, but only at the focal point,

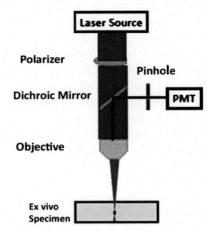

Confocal Microscopy

Fig. 6.3 Confocal microscopy setup. Confocal microscopy represents the natural evolution of epifluorescence techniques. This approach schematically takes advantage of the replacement of the fluorescence lamp with a laser source, increasing the excitation power of the system, and of the introduction of a pinhole before the detector, here represented by a photomultiplier (PMT), that acts as an optical diaphragm and avoids any contribution of useless photons, such as scattered photons, to the acquired image

limiting the photobleaching of near off-focus tissues [61] (Fig. 6.4).

Scope

The spot-focused excitation limits photobleaching of fluorescent markers and reduces photodamage, increasing the duration of experiments without bias induced by procedural damage. Moreover, near-infrared (NIR) excitation wavelengths allow deeper penetration into biological tissues and reduce light scattering.

Thus, by serially and rapidly scanning the sample in the x–y plane along the z axis, it is possible to compose a high-resolution 3D image, reducing photobleaching of the fluorophores, improving background discrimination, and minimizing photodamage to living tissue [62].

For these particular features, two-photon excitation microscopy is used to scan thick living tissue samples, such as brain slices and

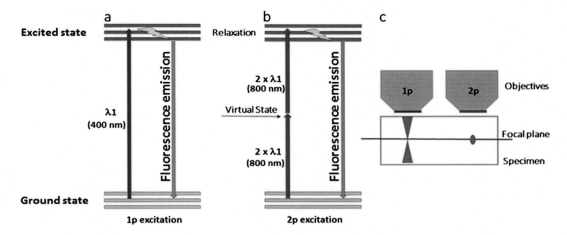

Fig. 6.4 Jablonski diagram. In (**a** and **b**), a fluorochrome emits light when an electron relaxes from an excited energy state to its ground state. The electron moves from the ground level to the excited level by absorbing one (**a**) or multiple (**b**) photons, an event that must occur at the same time and location (within about 15 fs), during the virtual state. (**c**) A layout showing the typical emission following one- or two-photon excitation. The scanning one-photon laser excites an entire column of sample, while the two-photon excitation excites only a small spot of sample. Two-photon excitation imaging has deep tissue penetration, little out-of-focal light absorption and least phototoxic effects

developing embryos, that would be difficult, if not impossible, to image with other microscopy techniques [63–67].

Technique Description

The basic principle of multiphoton excitation is a relatively old theoretical concept in quantum optics [61]. It was first proposed by Maria Göppert-Mayer while she was conducting her doctoral dissertation research in 1931 then observed experimentally some 30 years later, after the invention of pulsed ruby laser. Subsequently, the important work of Denk, Strickler, and Webb, published in *Science* in 1990, launched a new revolution in nonlinear optical microscopy, implementing multiphoton excitation processes into microscopy by combining a laser scanning microscope (scanning mirrors, PMT tube detection system) with a mode-locked laser that generated pulses of NIR light.

A crucial concept in explaining multiphoton processes is that, at high photon densities, two incident photons (if spatially and temporally overlapped) can be simultaneously absorbed by an electron of the molecule (i.e., the fluorophore), determining its excitation [68]. The molecule in the excited state has a high probability of emitting a photon during relaxation to the ground state, detectable as fluorescence emission. Moreover, since the energy of a photon is inversely proportional to its wavelength, the two absorbed photons must have a wavelength about twice that required for single-photon excitation (Fig. 6.4).

The introduction of high-power mode-locked pulsed lasers has enabled features that can generate high-photon densities (a photon concentration approximately a million times that required to generate the same number of one-photon absorptions) during pulse peaks. To date, tunable mode-locked titanium–sapphire lasers with high repetition rates (typically 80–90 MHz) and an ultrashort pulse duration (<200 fs) are typically used as NIR sources in multiphoton excitation imaging. The laser light generated by the mode-locked pulsed lasers can be focused by the microscope objective to such a limited focal volume that intensity is sufficient to generate appreciable excitation.

The resulting emission is identical to that achieved following a conventional fluorescence experiment and can be detected by placing an

2p Microscopy

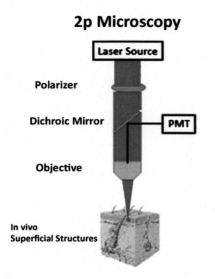

Fig. 6.5 Two-photon microscopy setup. Two-photon setup is very similar to that of the epifluorescence microscope with the exception of the laser source, which is generally based on a mode-locked titanium–sapphire laser. It is able to provide a high density of photons in a short time, and optical pathways are congruent to the wavelength selected. Similar to microscope and confocal systems, the excitation photons emitted by the sample can be scattered. However, the probability of two photons being scattered to the same location and time is almost zero; consequently, a better signal-to-noise ratio is achieved without the use of a pinhole

external photon detection device as close as possible to the sample (Fig. 6.5).

Examples

Regarding human pathologies, with its intrinsic depth limits, two-photon microscopy has been applied in the characterization of microscopically superficial structures, mainly to analyze skin lesions. Recently, Masters and So compared the use of multi-photon excitation microscopy and confocal scanning microscopy for imaging human skin in vivo [69–73]. Multi-photon excitation is induced by an 80 MHz pulse train of femtosecond laser pulses at 780 nm wavelength. These features are employed to excite intrinsic fluorophores in the skin, such as the reduced pyridine nucleotides (NAD(P)H) in the epidermis, a marker of cellular oxidative metabolism, and the collagen and elastin fibers in the dermis.

Advanced Microscopy Techniques

Introduction

We have previously noted that multiphoton fluorescence microscopy represents the state of the art for in vivo imaging of cells and tissues as it minimizes photobleaching and therefore photodamage of specimens. Moreover, we have shown that this advanced technique may be applied to human and skin pathologies, employing the nontoxic nature of two-photon excitation for skin autofluorescence investigation.

Although this technique represents the first choice for imaging living tissues, classic two-photon microscopy has generally been limited to superficial areas, providing good resolution to a depth of about ~500–700 μm. This phenomenon is due to photon scattering, which limits the optical penetration of light within tissues. To image cells in deeper areas, an adaptation of this technique has recently been created: in vivo optical microendoscopy [74, 75]. This approach can overcome this depth limit through the use of needlelike micro-optical probes and can involve one- or two-photon fluorescence excitation.

It is possible to customize the optical setups so that microendoscope probes of different lengths and diameters could be arranged to image nearby tissue in vivo and in a noninvasive manner. This would allow clinicians to follow the microscopic evolution/drug response of a lesion over time, without surgical excision, and to dynamically observe tissues in their physiological environment [64, 76] (Fig. 6.6).

Scope

The introduction of new research tools with fiber-based devices with smaller diameters (ranging from 350 to 1000 mm in diameter) and micron-scale resolution has seen "microendoscope fluorescence imaging" become increasingly versatile over the last decade, analyzing deep structures that have previously been inaccessible to microscopy [77].

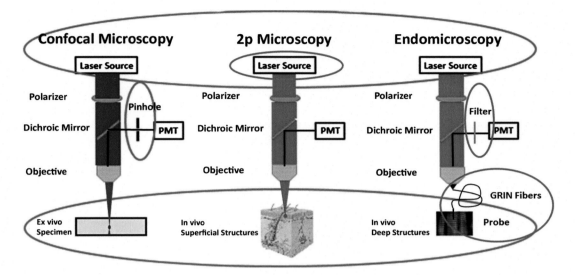

Fig. 6.6 Microendoscopy setup. The layout schematizes the technical evolution of microscope from confocal to two-photon to microendoscopy design. As for two-photon microscopy, a titanium–sapphire laser emits about 100-fs pulses of infrared excitation light. The laser beam is driven at the objective, where it is focused through the gradient refractive index (GRIN) optical fibers to a focal spot just above the external face of the endoscope probe, inserted also far from the microscope body

Recent devices are based on several micro-lenses of the gradient refractive index (GRIN) that act like optical fibers to acquire images of the specimen and project it at a distance.

The possibility of imaging sites that conventional light microscopy cannot access, of performing longitudinal observations and microscopic follow-up of lesions and therapeutic effects, and of developing minimally invasive clinical diagnostic tests has strengthened research in fiber-optic imaging [78, 79].

Although fluorescence microendoscopy is in its infancy, widespread applications are possible in the future, such as minimally invasive microscopic characterization of a lesion or a therapy response and extemporaneous pathological evaluation during surgery but before an excision is made [79, 80].

Technique Description

Microendoscopes are available in different optical setups, according to excitation source, probe, objective, and, primarily, target [74].

Nearly any upright microscope arranged for in vivo imaging could be adapted for microendoscopy. In terms of the body of the microscope and the microendoscope probe working together, two options are available: the microendoscope probe can be directly linked to the target specimen or to the body of the microscope.

A microendoscope probe is made with two serial optical components: an infinity micro-objective near the specimen that focuses excitation light and subsequently collects emitted fluorescence from the sample, and a micro-optical relay lens that focuses the emission photons to the upright microscope's objective lens.

Microendoscope probes can be customized according to specific applications and tissue targets by modifying optical parameters such as the diameter, length, or magnification to achieve selected spatial resolution and field of view.

The diameter can vary from 0.35 to 2.8 mm without affecting resolution or magnification. Wider probes generally have broader fields of view and are less fragile. However, their positioning within the sample can be more invasive.

The length of the microendoscope can also vary according to the depth of the tissue target to be imaged and the surgical preparation.

Moreover, the length of the probe can affect spatial resolution for the accumulation of optical distortions across the light pathway.

Finally, magnification can also be customized according to the field of view and the diameter of the microendoscope probe. Generally, the magnification of a 10× objective should be sufficient to cover the top surface of a probe with a diameter of 1 mm.

Examples

Regarding in vivo human pathologies, Cromie et al. recently applied this technique in the functional analysis of muscles and sarcomere structure [81]. In their experiment, they used an excitation wavelength of 960 nm to maximize the image signal. Briefly, a 500-μm diameter GRIN probe was inserted into the proximal third of the human extensor carpi radialis brevis muscle belly, and sarcomere lengths were measured with the body in different postures [81, 82].

Advanced Molecular Imaging

Introduction

The definition of molecular imaging given by the Society of Nuclear Medicine is "the visualization, characterization and measurement of biological processes at the molecular and cellular level in humans and other living systems" [83, 84].

More specifically, molecular imaging probes the molecular abnormalities of diseases to allow earlier detection, monitoring of disease progression, and assessment of treatments. It represents the next revolution in medical imaging, consisting of a multidisciplinary approach to improve diagnostic accuracy and sensitivity by means of an in vivo analogue of immunocytochemistry or in situ hybridization [85].

Combining multimodality imaging systems with molecular target-specific tracers allows increased individualized accuracy in diagnosis, treatment response prediction, and evaluation as well as prognosis [86, 87].

This revolution has been sustained by the introduction of hybrid imaging systems, in which morphological imaging modalities, such as computed tomography (CT) and MRI, are complemented by functional imaging modalities such as PET. Moreover, the increasing understanding of cellular and molecular events in the various signal transduction pathways and the development of highly selective probes have enabled this improvement.

Because molecules themselves are obviously too small to be imaged directly with noninvasive techniques, specific and sensitive site-targeted contrast agents are typically employed as beacons to depict epitopes of interest.

Carrier moieties, such as nanoparticles (liposomes or emulsions), dendrimers, viral constructs, buckyballs, or various polymers, can be loaded with large levels of imaging agents such as paramagnetic or superparamagnetic metals, optically active compounds (e.g., fluorescent molecules), or radionuclides, meaning they can be detected with standard imaging equipment. In the case of ultrasound (US) imaging, the intrinsic physical properties of the carrier agents themselves (density and compressibility) establish the means for detection. For certain constructs, such as liquid perfluorocarbon nanoparticles, considerable flexibility exists to utilize any or all imaging modalities.

As specified above, the molecular tracer employed in a specific study must be detectable by and thus labeled specifically for a particular diagnostic technique (CT, MR, US PET, single-photon emission computed tomography [SPECT]). As such, traditional radiology and CT use contrast media with various densities, such as iodinated compounds; MR uses paramagnetic and/or super-paramagnetic agents; ultrasonography involves contrast agents with different degrees of echogenicity with respect to the surrounding soft tissues, such as microbubbles; and nuclear medicine uses radionuclides that emit radiation detectable from outside the body.

Based on the probes used, molecular imaging can be classified into "direct" and "indirect" imaging approaches: direct imaging involves signal-generating moieties targeted to endogenous molecules of diseased tissue; indirect imaging utilizes reporter genes to report on activities of artificially introduced genes/promoters in the cells/tissues in living subjects [87].

Among the different imaging techniques, nuclear medicine, ultrasonography, and, in recent years, also MRI, have represented good instrumental candidates for molecular imaging, both for diagnosis and for target-specific treatment, employing mainly direct imaging approaches.

Scope

This section aims to provide the reader with an introductory overview of the main advanced diagnostic imaging fields (nuclear medicine, ultrasonography, and MR) related to molecular targeting. After discussing the molecular aspects of each imaging modality, we focus our attention on the power of multimodality integration.

Technique Description

Nuclear Medicine and Molecular Imaging

In terms of diagnosing and staging oncologic diseases, the identification of sentinel lymph nodes provides surgeons, oncologists, and referring physicians with vital information [83]. Lymphatic metastasis is an important prognostic factor in malignancies, and most tumors are classified according to the TNM (tumor, node, metastasis) staging system, which includes lymph node staging [88].

The long-standing mode of lymphatic mapping has been single or dual use of Tc-99 m sulfur colloid and isosulfan blue dye, which has inherent issues related to cost and a potential for allergic reaction [89].

Modern lymphoscintigraphy based on target-specific molecular imaging involves newcomer lymph node-specific tracers, such as Tc-99 m tilmanocept, or Tc-99 m nano-colloid, for the best binding to and higher detection of lymph nodes and faster washout from injection site to the sentinel nodes, minimizing complications.

The tilmanocept employs its natural affinity for the CD206 mannose receptor in lymph node targeting and mapping, while the nano-colloid uses the albumin-based imaging agent. However, it is important to realize that these tracers help to map the lymphatic net, identifying putative tumor-draining lymph nodes, but they are not tumor specific. Therefore, further efforts must be made to differentiate metastatic nodes from reactive nodes.

Most nuclear imaging applications of molecular imaging use "direct" imaging. For example, somatostatin-receptor imaging is used for the detection of neuroendocrine tumors, and fluorodeoxyglucose (FDG) imaging is used to characterize disease states (Fig. 6.7). Another example of direct imaging is the use of the molecular probe 99mTc-Annexin V to image the process of apoptosis. This is a very interesting tool for determining the efficacy of chemotherapy in patients with known cancer and the death of cancerous cells.

Another exciting molecular imaging agent is Zevalin®, a US FDA-approved radioimmunotherapy agent used in patients with rituximab-refractory follicular non-Hodgkin's lymphoma (NHL). This probe can be labeled with 111 In for imaging or with 90Y for treatment, with a response rate of about 74 % in these patients and no significant adverse events reported.

Similarly, radium-223 dichloride is a promising molecular-targeted treatment for patients with advanced tumors such as prostate cancer with bone metastasis. These patients, who generally have a poor prognosis, could be treated with radium-223 dichloride, a targeted radioisotope that concentrates specifically in bone metastases and releases alpha particles that kill tumoral cells, reducing pain and increasing survival rates.

Other efforts are being made to develop probes against direct targets to differentiate normal and diseased tissues, necessary for improved disease management. Some well-known examples are radiolabeled Herceptin® (a monoclonal antibody

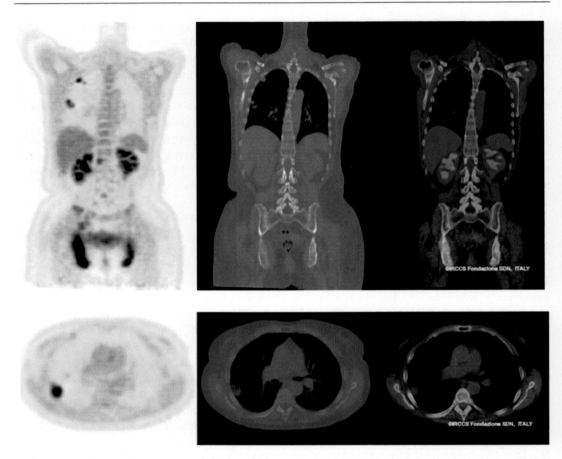

Fig. 6.7 Simultaneous computed tomography (CT)/positron emission tomography (PET) multimodal examination with administration of the 18 F-deoxyglucose (FDG) radiotracer. *Top*: Coronal views of (from *left* to *right*) PET, CT, and PET—CT fusion. *Bottom*: Axial views of (from *left* to *right*) PET, CT, and PET—CT fusion. Courtesy of IRCCS Fondazione SDN, Naples, Italy

against Her2Neu receptors, which is often overexpressed in breast cancer) or Avastin® (a monoclonal antibody generated against vascular endothelial growth factor [VEGF] receptor, required for neoangiogenesis).

Ultrasonography and Molecular Imaging

US is the most widely used cross-sectional imaging modality worldwide [90]. US contrast agents (UCAs) can be used to improve imaging by introducing a material with different acoustic properties from that of tissues [91].

UCAs carrying targeting ligands on the particle surface, such as monoclonal antibodies, have been suggested as selective imaging agents for the detection and evaluation of intravascular pathology, including thrombosis, inflammation, ischemia–reperfusion injury, or neoangiogenesis. The design of targeted contrast particles can differ widely, encompassing a multilayer liposome, a liquid fluorocarbon particle, or a gas-filled microbubble. This represents the most common approach to US molecular imaging [92].

Microbubbles can be quantified in passive and active imaging approaches. In passive approaches, low acoustic power is used to observe the enhancement effects without disrupting the microbubbles. Conversely, the active approach instead uses a transient pulse of high acoustic power to destroy microbubbles and then observe them refilling into an area of interest during an infusion [93].

Some microbubbles are tissue specific (e.g., some show tropism for the reticuloendothelial system, probably through direct phagocytosis by the Kupffer cells in the liver and spleen), and this can also be exploited in a number of emerging applications. The phospholipid shell contrast agent AF0150 (Imavist; Alliance Pharmaceutical, San Diego, CA, USA) is one such agent.

However, one area in which functional methods are moving beyond the research arena and becoming established clinical tools is in the liver. Using microbubble US, the classic contrastographic pattern of different lesions detected by CT or MRI can also be highlighted by US, differentiating hemangiomas from liver dysplasia or cirrhosis.

Several strategies have been developed to promote the targeting of microbubble contrast agents to specific regions of disease. Potential ligands include antibodies, peptides, and polysaccharides. Most targeted UCAs are microbubbles, but other vehicles can be used, including acoustically active liposomes and perfluorocarbon emulsions.

Using antibodies to P- or E-selectin (or to cell-adhesion molecules such as intercellular adhesion molecule [ICAM]-1) conjugated to a phospholipid shelled microbubble, it is possible to specifically image inflammation sites. Lipid-based microbubble contrast agent conjugated of echistatin to the shell surface can be targeted to alfavbeta3, an integrin highly expressed by angiogenic endothelium.

MRX-408 or MRX-408A1 (ImaRx Inc., Tucson, AZ, USA) incorporate the Arg-Gly-Asp (RGD) peptide sequence (adherent to the receptors for fibrinogen and von Willebrand factor) in the lipid-shelled microbubble to selectively target thrombi.

Perfluorocarbon emulsion nanoparticles can be used as an efficacious UCA, combining the benefits of traditional gas-encapsulated microbubbles and liposomes.

Magnetic Resonance and Molecular Imaging

Molecular imaging based on MRI has significant advantages in clinical diagnosis and prognosis [94]. With respect to other conventional modalities, MRI offers superior spatial resolution without depth limitation, exquisite soft tissue contrast, clinical availability, and avoids ionizing radiation [95, 96] (Fig. 6.8).

For paramagnetic agents, it is important that the longitudinal relaxivity per molecular binding site for the complex is maximized, allowing contrast enhancement with very small numbers of paramagnetic particles. For paramagnetic perfluorocarbon nanoparticles, for example, particle-based relaxivities (or "unit signal strength") are the highest reported to date in the literature, providing a signal detectable at local concentrations in the picomolar range [97].

Paramagnetic polymerized liposomes and liquid perfluorocarbon nanoparticle emulsions targeted to neovascular integrins alfavbeta3 have been used to image experimental tumor angiogenesis. Indeed, liquid perfluorocarbon nanoparticles were the first example of molecular targeting agents broadly useful for MRI of thrombi by means of incorporating antibody ligands directed against cross-linked fibrin.

Stem-cell labeling with magneto-dendrimers enables MRI for detection and precise localization after therapeutic injection [97–100].

Other so-called smart agents employ indirect imaging; they are designed to take up residence in all cells of the body but to be activated only by specific enzymes that are expressed in the cell under certain pathological states or by the protein products (enzymes) of reporter genes after therapeutic transfection.

Superparamagnetic iron oxide (SPIO) particles, such as ferumoxides (Feridex, Bayer HealthCare), are MRI contrast agents that endow the cells of interest with straightforward hypo-intense contrast enhancement after proper labeling. This SPIO formulation is the only pharmaceutical-grade MRI contrast agent that has been used for clinical cell tracking of labeled T cells to a site of

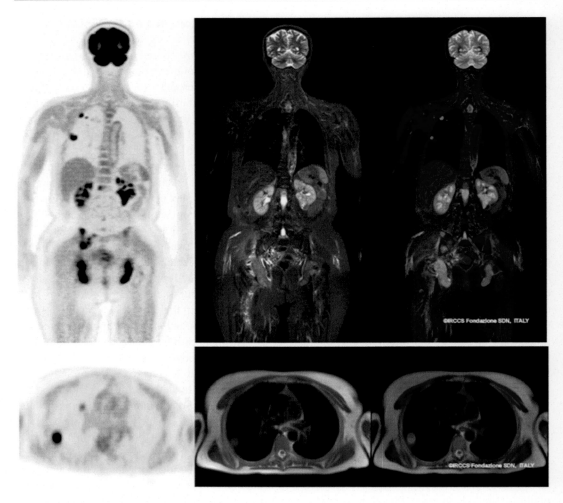

Fig. 6.8 Simultaneous magnetic resonance (MR)/positron emission tomography (PET) multimodal examination with administration of 18 F-deoxyglucose (FDG) radiotracer. *Top*: Coronal views of (from *left* to *right*) PET, MR, and PET—MR fusion. *Bottom*: axial views of (from *left* to *right*) PET, MR, and PET—MR fusion. Courtesy of IRCCS Fondazione SDN, Naples, Italy

inflammation, or paramagnetically labeled stem cells to damaged tissues for "cell therapy."

Hybrid Molecular Imaging

Although single imaging modality has been applied in a variety of imaging fields, it is constrained by the limitation that it cannot offer all the required information. Eventually, this challenge has led to the appearance of the multimodal imaging era in biomedical applications. Various forms of hybrid imaging systems that combine two or more imaging modalities have

been developed to provide more precise detection of disease and abnormal functions for clinical application. In particular, studies of PET/MR dual modality have revealed them to be powerful research tools in terms of simultaneous anatomical and functional image acquisition (Figs. 6.7 and 6.8).

Several authors have demonstrated that a magnetic imaging sensor labeled with a PET imaging probe (124I-labeled MnMEIO nanoparticle) was effective for the tracking of sentinel lymph nodes [101].

As mentioned above, RGD peptides already known as potential cancer-targeting ligands were successfully applied in multimodal imaging for cancer detection, by means of DOTA chelating agents (64Cu-DOTA-IO-RGD particle). Well-matched radiopharmaceuticals, including F-18 FDG, or specific trackers such as C-11 acetate and C-11 choline, greatly improve the specificity of PET/MR.

Lessons Learned

The target-specific molecular probe is a crucial step in the development of a diagnostic and therapeutic workflow addressing personalized medicine.

The identification of specific pathogenic markers and the possibility of detecting them in vivo are essential recipes for the early diagnosis and staging of disease.

The integration of the findings carried out by each modality of hybrid systems enables a reduction in acquisition time, improving diagnostic accuracy.

References

1. Arrebola F, Cañizares J, Cubero MA, Crespo PV, Warley A, Fernández-Segura E. Biphasic behavior of changes in elemental composition during staurosporine-induced apoptosis. Apoptosis. 2005;10(6):1317–31.
2. Zhang M, Methot D, Poppa V, et al. Cardiomyocyte grafting for CardiacRepair: graft cell death and anti-DeathStrategies. J Mol Cell Cardiol. 2001;33:907–21.
3. Lucic V, Rigort A, Baumeister W. Cryo-electron tomography: the challenge of doing structural biology in situ. J Cell Biol. 2013;202(3):407–19.
4. Millonig G, Marinozzi V. Fixation and embedding in electron microscopy. Adv Optical Electron Microsc. 1968;2:251.
5. Stein O, Stein Y. Light and electron microscopic radioautography of lipids: techniques and biological applications. Adv Lipid Res. 1971;9:1–72.
6. Mizuhira V, Futaesaku Y. New fixation method for biological membranes using tannic acids. Acta Histochem Cytochem. 1972;5:233–6.
7. Hirsch JG, Fedorko ME. Ultrastructure of human leukocytes after simultaneous fixation with glutaraldehyde and osmium tetroxide and "postfixation" in uranyl acetate. J Cell Biol. 1968;38:615–27.
8. Silva MT, Guerra FC, Magalhaes MM. The fixative action of uranyl acetate in electron microscopy. Experientia. 1968;24:1074.
9. Mollenhauer HH. Artifacts caused by dehydration and epoxy embedding in transmission electron microscopy. Microsc Res Tech. 1993;26:496–512.
10. Tokuyasu KT. A technique for ultracryotomy of cell suspensions and tissues. J Cell Biol. 1973;57:551–65.
11. Griffiths G, McDowall A, Back R, Dubochet J. On the preparation of cryosections for immunocyto-chemistry. J Ultrastruct Res. 1984;89:65–78.
12. Slot JW, Geuze HJ. Cryosectioning and immunolabeling. Nat Protoc. 2007;2:2480–91.
13. Herpers B, Xanthakis D, Rabouille C. ISH-IEM: a sensitive method to detect endogenous mRNAs at the ultrastructural level. Nat Protoc. 2010;5:678–87.
14. Müller HR. Freeze-drying as a fixation technic for plant cells. J Ultrastruct Res. 1957;1:109–37.
15. Steere RL. Electron microscopy of structural detail in frozen biological specimens. J Biophys Biochem Cytol. 1957;3:45–60.
16. Moor H, Muhlethaler K, Waldner H, Frey-Wyssling A. A new freezing ultramicrotome. J Biophys Biochem Cytol. 1961;10:1–13.
17. Braet F, De Zanger R, Wisse E. Drying cells for SEM, AFM and TEM by hexamethyldisilazane: a study on hepatic endothelial cells. J Microsc. 1997;186:84–8713.
18. Bray DF, Bagu J, Koegler P. Comparison of hexamethyldisilazane (HMDS), Peldri II, and critical-point drying methods for scanning electron microscopy of biological specimens. Microsc Res Tech. 1993;26:489–95.
19. Moor H. Theory and practice of high pressure freezing. In: Steinbrecht RA, Zierold K, editors. Cryotechniques in biological electron microscopy. Berlin: Springer; 1987. p. 175–91.
20. Allison DP, Daw CS, Rorvik MC. The construction and operation of a simple inexpensive slam freezing device for electron microscopy. J Microsc. 1987;147:103–8.
21. Dubochet J. The physics of rapid cooling and its implications for cryoimmobilization of cells. Methods Cell Biol. 2007;79:7–21.
22. Escaig J. New instruments which facilitate rapid freezing at 83 K and 6 K. J Microsc. 1982;126:221–9.
23. Meryman HT. Cryopreservation of living cells: principles and practice. Transfusion. 2007;47:935–45.
24. De Carlo S. Plunge freezing (Holey Carbon Method). In: Cavelier A, Spehner D, Humbel BM, editors. Handbook of cryo-preparation methods for electron microscopy. Boca Raton, FL: CRC Press; 2009. p. 49–68.

25. Galway ME, Heckman Jr JW, Hyde GJ, Fowke LC. Advances in high-pressure and plunge-freeze fixation. Methods Cell Biol. 1995;49:3–19.

26. Nitta K, Kaneko Y. Simple plunge freezing applied to plant tissues for capturing the ultrastructure close to the living state. J Electron Microsc (Tokyo). 2004;53:677–80.

27. Richter T, Biel SS, Sattler M, Wenck H, Wittern KP, Wiesendanger R, Wepf R. Pros and cons: cryo-electron microscopic evaluation of block faces versus cryo-sections from frozen-hydrated skin specimens prepared by different techniques. J Microsc. 2007;225:201–7.

28. Riehle U, Hoechli M. The theory and technique of high pressure freezing. In: Benedetti EL, Favard P, editors. Freeze etching techniques and applications. Paris: SociétéFrançaise de MicroscopieElectronique; 1973. p. 31–61.

29. Brown E, Mantell J, Carter DA, Tilly G, Verkate B. Studying intracellular transport using high pressure freezing and correlative light electron microscopy. Semin Cell Dev Biol. 2009;20:910–9.

30. Claeys M, Vanhecke D, Couvreur M, Tytgat T, Coomans A, Borgonie G. High-pressure freezing and freeze substitution of gravid Caenorhabditis elegans (Nematoda: Rhabditida) for transmission electron microscopy. Nematology. 2004;6:319–27.

31. Hohenberg H, Tobler M, Muller M. High-pressure freezing of tissue obtained by fine-needle biopsy. J Microsc. 1996;183:133–9.

32. Vanhecke D, Graber W, Herrmann G, Al-Amoudi A, Eggli P, Studer D. A rapid microbiopsy system to improve the preservation of biological samples prior to high-pressure freezing. 2003. J Microsc.

33. Shanbhag SR, Park SK, Pikielny CW, Steinbrecht RA. Gustatory organs of drosophila melanogaster: the structure and expression of the putative odorant-binding protein PBPRP2. Cell Tissue Res. 2001;304:423–37.

34. Wang L, Humbel BM, Roubos EW. High-pressure freezing followed by cryosubstitution as a tool for preserving high-quality ultrastructure and immunoreactivity in the Xenopuslaevis pituitary gland. Brain Res Brain Res Protoc. 2005;15:155–63.

35. Moor H, Mühletaler K. Fine structure in frozen-etched yeast cells. J Cell Biol. 1963;17:609–28.

36. Van Harreveld A, Crowell J. Electron microscopy after rapid freezing on a metal surface and substitution Wxation. Anat Rec. 1964;149:381–5.

37. Al-Amoudi A, Chang JJ, Leforestier A, McDowall A, Salamin LM, Norlen LP, Richter K, Blanc NS, Studer D, Dubochet J. Cryo-electron microscopy of vitreous sections. EMBO J. 2004;23:3583.

38. Dubochet J, McDowall AW, Menge B, Schmid EN, Lickfeld KG. Electron microscopy of frozen-hydrated bacteria. J Bacteriol. 1983;155:381–90.

39. Branton D. Freeze-etching studies of membrane structure. Philos Trans R Soc Lond B Biol Sci. 1971;261:133–8.

40. Heuser JE, Reese TS, Dennis MJ, Jan Y, Jan L, Evans L. Synaptic vesicle exocytosis captured by quick freezing and correlated with quantal transmitter release.J. Cell Biol. 1979;81:275–300.

41. Guerquin-Kern JL, Wu TD, Quintana C, Croisy A. Progress in analytical imaging of the cell by dynamic secondary ion mass spectrometry (SIMS microscopy). Biochim Biophys Acta. 2005;1724:228–38.

42. Lucic V, Forster F, Baumeister W. Structural studies by electron tomography: from cells to molecules. Annu Rev Biochem. 2005;74:833–65.

43. Lucic V, Leis A, Baumeister W. Cryo-electron tomography of cells: connecting structure and function. Histochem Cell Biol. 2008;130:185–96.

44. Eltsov M, Maclellan KM, Maeshima K, Frangakis AS, Dubochet J. Analysis of cryo-electron microscopy images does not support the existence of 30-nm chromatin fibers in mitotic chromosomes in situ. Proc Natl Acad Sci U S A. 2008;105:19732–7.

45. Salje J, Zuber B, Löwe J. Electron cryomicroscopy of E. coli reveals filament bundles involved in plasmid DNA segregation. Science. 2009;323:509–12.

46. Zuber B, Chami M, Houssin C, Dubochet J, Griffiths G, Daffé M. Direct visualization of the outer membrane of mycobacteria and corynebacteriain their native state.J. Bacteriology. 2008;190:5672–80.

47. Bleck CK, Merz A, Gutierrez MG, Walther P, Dubochet J, Zuber B, Griffiths G. Comparison of different methods for thin section EM analysis of Mycobacterium smegmatis. J Microsc. 2010;237:23–38.

48. Koning RI, Koster KAJ. Cryo-electron tomography in biology and medicine. Ann Anat. 2009;191:427–45.

49. Gilbert P. Iterative methods for the three dimensional reconstruction of an object from projections. J Theor Biol. 1972;36:105–17.

50. Jonic S, Sorzano COS, Boisset N. Comparison of single-particle analysis and electron tomography approaches: an overview. J Microsc. 2008;232:562–79.

51. Koster AJ, Klumperman J. Electron microscopy in cell biology: integrating structure and function. Nat Rev Mol Cell Biol. 2003;4(Suppl):SS6–10.

52. Garvalov BK, Zuber B, Bouchet-Marquis C, Kudryashev M, Gruska M, Beck M, Leis A, Frischknecht F, Bradke F, Baumeister W, et al. Luminal particles within cellular microtubules.J. Cell Biol. 2006;174:759–65.

53. Braet F, Wisse E, Bomans P, Frederik P, Geerts W, Koster A, Soon L, Ringer S. Contribution of high-resolution correlative imaging techniques in the study of the liver sieve in three-dimensions. Microsc Res Tech. 2007;70:230–42.

54. Nickell S, Kofler C, Leis AP, Baumeister W. A visual approach to proteomics. Nat Rev Mol Cell Biol. 2006;7:225–30.

55. Humbel BM, de Jong MD, Müller WH, Verkleij AJ. Pre-embedding immunolabeling for electron microscopy: an evaluation of permeabilization methods and markers. Microsc Res Tech. 1998;42:43–58.

56. http://www.olympusmicro.com/

57. http://www.microscopyu.com/

58. Denk WJ, Strickler JP, Webb WW. Two-photon laser scanning fluorescence microscopy. Science. 1990;248:73–6.

59. Zipfel WR, Williams RM, Christie R, et al. Live tissue intrinsic emission microscopy using multiphoton-excited native fluorescence and second harmonic generation. Proc Natl Acad Sci U S A. 2003;100(12):7075–80.

60. Konig K, Riemann I. High-resolution multiphoton tomography of human skin with subcellular spatial resolution and picosecond time resolution. J Biomed Opt. 2003;8(3):432–9.

61. Svoboda K, Yasuda R. Principles of two-photon excitation microscopy and its applications to neuroscience. Neuron. 2006 Jun 15;50(6):823–39.

62. Wang BG, Konig K, Halbhuber KJ. Two-photon microscopy of deep intravital tissues and its merits in clinical research. J Microsc. 2010;238(Pt 1):1–20.

63. Williams RM, Zipfel WR, Webb WW. Multiphoton microscopy in biological research. Curr Opin Chem Biol. 2001;5(5):603–7.

64. Helmchen F, Denk W. Deep tissue two-photon microscopy. Nat Methods. 2005;2(12):932–40.

65. Marcello L, Cavaliere C, Colangelo AM, Bianco MR, Cirillo G, Alberghina L, Papa M. Remodelling of supraspinal neuroglial network in neuropathic pain is featured by a reactive gliosis of the nociceptive amygdala. Eur J Pain. 2013 Jul;17(6):799–810.

66. Squirrell JM, Wokosin DL, White JG, Bavister BD. Long- term two-photon fluorescence imaging of mammalian embryos without compromising viability. Nat Biotechnol. 1999;17:763–7.

67. Maggio N, Cavaliere C, Papa M, Blatt I, Chapman J, Segal M. Thrombin regulation of synaptic transmission: implications for seizure onset. Neurobiol Dis. 2013 Feb;50:171–7.

68. Campagnola PJ, Loew LM. Second-harmonic imaging microscopy for visualizing biomolecular arrays in cells, tissues and organisms. Nat Biotechnol. 2003;21(11):1356–60.

69. Guo Y, Savage HE, Liu F, Schantz SP, Ho PP, Alfano RR. Subsurface tumor progression investigated by non-invasive optical second harmonic tomography. Proc Natl Acad Sci U S A. 1999;96(19):10854–6.

70. Masters BR, So PTC. Multi-photon excitation microscopy and confocal microscopy imaging of in vivo human skin: a comparison. Micros Microanal. 1999;5:282–9.

71. Masters BR, So PTC, Gratton E. Optical biopsy of in vivo human skin: multiphoton excitation microscopy. Lasers Med Sci. 1998;13:196–203.

72. Schenke-Layland K, Riemann I, Damour O, Stock UA, Konig K. Two-photon microscopes and in vivo multiphoton tomographs—Powerful diagnostic tools for tissue engineering and drug delivery. Adv Drug Deliv Rev. 2006;58:878–96.

73. Cirillo G, De Luca D, Papa M. Calcium imaging of living astrocytes in the mouse spinal cord following sensory stimulation. Neural Plast. 2012;2012:425818. doi:10.1155/2012/425817.

74. Mehta AD, Jung JC, Flusberg BA, Schnitzer MJ. Fiber optic in vivo imaging in the mammalian nervous system. Curr Opin Neurobiol. 2004;14:617–27.

75. Llewellyn ME, Barretto RP, Delp SL, Schnitzer MJ. Minimally invasive high-speed imaging of sarcomere contractile dynamics in mice and humans. Nature. 2007;454:784–7.

76. Wilt BA, Burns LD, Wei Ho ET, Ghosh KK, Mukamel EA, Schnitzer MJ. Advances in light microscopy for neuroscience. Annu Rev Neurosci. 2009;32:435–506.

77. Barretto RP, Ko TH, Jung JC, Wang TJ, Capps G, Waters AC, Ziv Y, Attardo A, Recht L, Schnitzer MJ. Time- lapse imaging of disease progression in deep brain areas using fluorescence microendoscopy. 2010.

78. Flusberg BA, Cocker ED, Piyawattanametha W, Jung JC, Cheung EL, Schnitzer MJ. Fiber-optic fluorescence imaging. Nat Methods. 2005;2:941–50.

79. Delaney PM, King RG, Lambert JR, Harris MR. Fibre optic confocal imaging (FOCI) for subsurface microscopy of the colon in vivo. J Anat. 1994;184:157–60.

80. Kiesslich R, et al. Confocal laser endoscopy for diagnosing intraepithelial neoplasias and colorectal cancer in vivo. Gastroenterology. 2004;127:706–13.

81. Cromie MJ, Sanchez GN, Schnitzer MJ, Delp SL. Sarcomere Lenghts in human extensor carpi radialis brevis measured by microendoscopy. Muscle Nerve. 2013;48(2):286–92.

82. Swindle LD, Thomas SG, Freeman M, Delaney PM. View of normal human skin in vivo as observed using fluorescent fiber-optic confocal microscopic imaging. J Invest Dermatol. 2003;121:706–12.

83. Blasberg RG. Molecular imaging and cancer. Mol Cancer Ther. 2003;2:335–43.

84. Grassi R, Cavaliere C, Cozzolino S, Mansi L, Cirillo S, Tedeschi G, Franchi R, Russo P, Cornacchia S, Rotondo A. Small animal imaging facility: new perspectives for the radiologist. Radiol Med. 2009;114:152–67.

85. Berritto D, Somma F, Landi N, Cavaliere C, Corona M, Russo S, Fulciniti F, Cappabianca S, Rotondo A, Grassi R. Seven-Tesla micro-MRI in early detection of acute arterial ischaemia: evolution of findings in an in vivo rat model. Radiol Med. 2011;116:829–41.

86. Doubrovin M, Serganova I, Mayer-Kuckuk P, et al. Multimodality in vivo molecular-genetic imaging. Bioconjug Chem. 2004;15:1376–87.

87. Luker GD, Piwnica-Worms D. Molecular imaging in vivo with PET and SPECT. Acad Radiol. 2001;8:4–14.

88. Stumpe KD, Urbinelli M, Steinert HC, et al. Whole body positron emission tomography using fluorodeoxyglucose for staging of lymphoma: effectiveness and comparison with computed tomography. Eur J Nucl Med. 1998;25:721–7.

89. Liang HD, Blomley MJ. The role of ultrasound in molecular imaging. Br J Radiol. 2003;76 suppl 2: S140–50.

90. Lindner JR. Molecular imaging with contrast ultrasound and targeted microbubbles. J Nucl Cardiol. 2004;11:215–21.

91. Unnikrishnan S, Klibanov AL. Microbubbles as ultrasound contrast agents for molecular imaging: preparation and application. AJR. 2012;199:292–9.

92. Klibanov AL, Rychak JJ, Yang WC, Alikhani S, Li B, Acton S, Lindner JR, Ley K, Kaul S. Targeted ultrasound contrast agent for molecular imaging of inflammation in high-shear flow. Contrast Media Mol Imaging. 2006;1:259–66.

93. Pace L, Nicolai E, Aiello M, Catalano OA, Salvatore M. Whole-body PET/MRI in oncology: current status and clinical applications. Clin Trans Imaging. 2013;1:31–44.

94. Rudin M, Weissleder R. Molecular imaging in drug discovery and development. Nat Rev Drug Discov. 2003;2:123–31.

95. Weissleder R. Molecular imaging: exploring the next frontier. Radiology. 1999;212:609–14.

96. Klerkx WM, Bax L, Veldhuis WB, Heintz APM, Mali WPTM, Peeters PHM, Moons KGM. Detection of lymph node metastases by gadolinium-enhanced magnetic resonance imaging: systematic review and meta-analysis. J Natl Cancer Inst. 2010;102:244–53.

97. Bulte JWM. In vivo MRI cell tracking: clinical studies. AJR. 2009;193:314–25.

98. Hwang DW, Youn H, Lee DS. Molecular imaging using PET/MRI particle. Open Nucl Med J. 2010;2:186–91.

99. Kamaly N, Miller AD. Paramagnetic liposome nanoparticles for cellular and tumour imaging. Int J Mol Sci. 2010;11:1759–76.

100. Tirino V, Desiderio V, d'Aquino R, De Francesco F, Pirozzi G, Graziano A, Galderisi U, Cavaliere C, De Rosa A, Papaccio G, Giordano A. Detection and characterization of CD133+ cancer stem cells in human solid tumours. PLoS One. 2008;3(10), e3469.

101. Brindle KM. Molecular imaging using magnetic resonance: new tools for the development of tumour therapy. Br J Radiol. 2003;76 suppl 2:S111–7.

Part III

Diagnostic Imaging and Pathology

Diagnostic Imaging and Pathology

7

Luigi Mansi, Vincenzo Cuccurullo, and Roberto Grassi

Introduction

This chapter serves as an introduction to the following sections concerning diagnostic imaging and its relationship with pathology.

- It starts with a general premise discussing how, despite being the gold standard in the traditional diagnostic scenario, pathology has some limitations, some of which can be overcome by a closer interaction with diagnostic imaging.
- The scope of this introductory chapter is to analyze how to optimize the relationship between diagnostic imaging and pathology.
- The third section focuses on the relationship between pathology and diagnostic imaging. In particular, we identify the most important fields in which diagnostic imaging can optimize pathology, either by improving its value or overcoming its limitations and mistakes.
- The fourth section discusses different categories, allowing a classification of diagnostic imaging techniques, noting the distinction between morphostructural and functional methods as most important.

- Major issues characterizing and differentiating morphostructural and functional techniques are discussed below.
- The chapter introduces the concept of molecular imaging as the most important part of diagnostic imaging in detecting and understanding the first stages of a disease. We also show that this capability is not connected only with recently introduced techniques but has been a constitutive part of nuclear medicine since it first began, many decades ago.
- The "lessons learned" focuses on the ability of diagnostic imaging to play a primary role in helping optimize pathology.
- The reference list includes the most important publications concerning the issue.

General Premise

In the traditional diagnostic universe, pathology is the gold standard, mainly because it provides the most accurate morphostructural information in clinical practice [1].

Nevertheless, results can be false-negative (FN) or, less frequently, false-positive (FP). False negatives may come about because of pathological characteristics, such as the lack of expression of a specific target, but more frequently are because of methodological issues, such as inappropriate techniques or a sampling

L. Mansi (✉) • V. Cuccurullo • R. Grassi
Sezione Scientifica di Radiodiagnostica, Radioterapia e Medicina Nucleare. Dipartimento Medico Chirurgico di Internistica Clinica e Sperimentale "F. MAGRASSI" e "A. LANZARA", Seconda Università degli Studi di Napoli, Naples, Italy
e-mail: luigi.mansi@unina2.it

© Springer Science+Business Media New York 2016
F.M. Sacerdoti et al. (eds.), *Advanced Imaging Techniques in Clinical Pathology*,
Current Clinical Pathology, DOI 10.1007/978-1-4939-3469-0_7

mistake. False positives occur when pathological procedures detect non-pathognomonic characteristics and thereby prevent a differential diagnosis [2].

In this scenario, accuracy could be increased with a wider and more precise pathological approach involving further samples, eventually guided by imaging, or by using multiple pathological techniques that can characterize different targets.

In clinical practice, the most important and frequent clinical question certainly involves the field of oncology. In this practical environment, routine first-line pathology procedures provide a response that ranges between the extremes "certainly normal" and "certainly malignant," but also includes probabilistic grades. Pathology alone cannot provide a correct final diagnosis; further contributions from different diagnostic approaches are therefore required [3].

Furthermore, modern medicine aims for "tailored medicine" that centers more on the individual patient than on the disease. Although current pathological procedures can certainly provide more information than ever before and can include prognostic content, pathology alone cannot answer all the questions clinicians and surgeons may have [4].

Pathology is certainly a primary and irreplaceable part of the overall diagnostic tree; however, it is not perfect and must be considered in the wider context, given its limits and the potential for mistakes.

A major issue for pathology is that it is impossible to obtain reliable information when the sample in question either does not represent or only partially represents the disease, which is possible in many conditions. For instance, where a biopsy is technically impossible (e.g., lesions are too deep, or invasive removal of a specimen is too dangerous); where sampling mistakes lead to incorrect analysis (e.g., analysis of a lesion that does not represent or shows the worst part of the malignancy); or where the sample is not fully or reliably evaluable because the tumor target is heterogeneous (e.g., different grades of malignancy in a single lesion, multiple neoplastic localizations with different targets and

consequently different biological behaviors). In terms of this last event, while pathology can be considered the gold standard for evaluating a single lesion, it is not practical in the staging or re-staging of cancer or diseases suspected as having spread since diagnosis. Furthermore, when lesions must be followed after therapeutic intervention, pathology is unable to analyze variations over time or evaluate therapeutic response in all localizations [5].

Scope

This introductory section aims to analyze how to optimize the relationship between diagnostic imaging (DI) and pathology.

To better understand the possible connections, we begin with those fields in which DI can optimize the effectiveness of pathology. We then delve more deeply into the field of DI, beginning with general classifications and mainly differentiating between morphostructural and functional techniques [5].

This chapter concludes with a discussion on how molecular imaging must be intended to optimize a new paradigm—personalized medicine— in which the focus is on the individual patient rather than the disease.

Diagnostic Imaging and Pathology

In the wider diagnostic scenario, DI can improve the effectiveness of pathology, which has recently been tasked with providing further prognostic and therapeutic information. Certainly, DI is pathology's best supporter (or, more precisely, a co-protagonist), with a range of important abilities [6].

Although DI also includes limitations and mistakes, it can also assist in the following ways:

1. Help localize all lesions through an evaluation guided by symptoms and/or a whole body analysis, essential in staging and re-staging of cancer and/or a range of benign diseases.

2. Guide biopsies, helping to individuate the most suspicious component in a single tumor, or the most accessible suspicious lesion, in presence of multifocal disease.
3. Guide surgery, through radionuclide (radioguided surgery) or radiological procedures, including metallic landmark or intra-surgical techniques.
4. Acquire supplemental information for pathology, enabling a more accurate differential diagnosis between benign and malignant diseases.
5. Enable correct staging (and re-staging), with the ability to detect primary neoplasms, metastases, and recurrence.
6. Add prognostic information complementary and/or different from that achievable by pathology.
7. Reliably recruit patients for a therapeutic strategy with the ability to also define "patho-physiological targets" that in vitro approaches are not able to evaluate. This situation represents a further limit for pathological analysis, which is unable to evaluate in vivo issues, such as biological barriers preventing a drug from reaching a "pathological" target.
8. Enable the evaluation of a therapeutic response in the primary tumor and metastases.

Classification of Diagnostic Imaging Techniques

While leaving a wider and deeper analysis to the specialized texts, here we present the most important characteristics of the major techniques and procedures in use. We also show, in the following subsections, particular applications of DI instruments used in humans and/or in the preclinical field to add to pathological information.

We can categorize DI techniques in many different ways.

The simplest and most effective classification, from the instructional viewpoint, is based on the individual signal/radiation generating the image.

In this context, we can first make a macroscopic distinction between techniques that are based on ionizing radiations (such as X-rays, gamma radiation, and positrons) and nonionizing radiation (NIR), the major representatives of which in clinical practice are ultrasounds (US) and magnetic resonance imaging (MRI) [7]. This separation is relevant in terms of calculating cost-effectiveness ratios, as diagnostic levels of ionizing radiation are connected with risks, which—although stochastic—are more critical in pregnant or pediatric subjects.

A further distinction can be made between planar (bidimensional) and tomographic (3D [three-dimensional]) techniques. In this context, the most important distinction must be within X-ray procedures, where we can distinguish between traditional radiology—typically bidimensional with or without a connection with a computer—and computed tomography (CT), which is a 3D computerized technique. The concept of 4D (four-dimensional) tomography has also been recently introduced, where the fourth temporal dimension individuates the presence of gating respiratory systems connected with hybrid machines.

With respect to the previous points, an ulterior general distinction that will disappear in the near future is between digital and analogical techniques, the latter individuating images acquired and represented without a computer connection. Almost all diagnostic machines are computerized, and a computer is mandatory for tomographic techniques; analogical procedures continue to exist only in traditional radiology, primarily for mammography (effective both as an analogical and a digital procedure) [12].

Morphostructural and Functional Techniques

From a clinical viewpoint, the most important distinction is between so-called morphostructural and functional techniques.

Morphostructural techniques are methods where the image represents differences in density. This approach may allow high spatial resolution, enabling millimetric (and in some cases also submillimetric) structures to be viewed; this is also an advantage in a locoregional analysis evaluating spatial anatomical relations. This category includes basic radiological procedures, i.e., performed without contrast media and/or not using more advanced technologies, such as those connected with Doppler in US and multiparametric approaches in MRI. With this limitation in mind, we can consider traditional radiology, CT, echography and, broadly, MRI to be morphostructural techniques. Morphological methods study anatomy and structural changes in healthy subjects and in patients, with pathology as the gold standard.

Functional procedures search for changes in concentration and/or in kinetic parameters to evaluate functional variations; as such, they define disease based on pathophysiological alterations. This category includes nuclear medicine, which is the only method that is exclusively functional. Moreover, both morphostructural and functional information may be obtained with traditional radiology and CT using contrast media, with US using Doppler or contrast media; and with MR, which is able to provide a wide series of functional images using spectroscopy, contrast media, and many sequences for the evaluation of different pathophysiological parameters [8].

Molecular Imaging

Living beings are made of molecules that are connected in a dynamic equilibrium called homeostasis [9]. Beginning with this definition, disease can be interpreted as an imbalance of the system; therefore, to provide the earliest possible diagnosis, it is the molecular level (nucleic acids, proteins, carbohydrates, etc.) that is the first to be investigated. It is possible to study molecular kinetics with molecular tracers, i.e., using "tracing" molecules following the same path of native molecules but to which a label detectable from the outside has been added. The nature of this label depends on the diagnostic technique, as

it must be able to create a signal-to-noise ratio suitable for the specific procedure [10, 11].

Traditional radiology and CT use contrast media that change density, such as iodinated compounds; MR uses paramagnetic and/or super-paramagnetic agents; US uses contrast agents with different degrees of echogenicity compared with surrounding soft tissues, such as microbubbles; and nuclear medicine uses radionuclides that emit radiation detectable from outside the body.

Both morphostructural and functional techniques have specific limitations. Functional methods are only of use in living beings and cannot correctly locate a lesion and/or define a structural alteration, which is essential in, for example, malformations [12]. Structural information may be less sensitive, also provided information that is less connected with prognosis and therapy. In the following section, we discuss the major technological improvements that have resulted from the introduction of so-called hybrid machines: where a nuclear medicine instrument (PET [positron emission tomography] or SPECT [single, photon emission computed tomography]) and a radiological tool (CT and—more recently and only currently in connection with PET—MRI) have been combined [13].

Lessons Learned

DI may have a primary role in optimizing pathology. Initially, it can locate pathological lesions, guide biopsy and surgery, and acquire supplemental pathological information, enabling more accurate diagnoses that differentiate between benign and malignant diseases. Together with in vivo morphostructural information, DI—when performed in conjunction with functional techniques—may not only increase the reliability of diagnosis, staging, or restaging but also contribute to prognosis, better defining the correct therapeutic approach. In terms of this latter point, DI may also enable the recruitment of patients for a therapeutic strategy based on "pathophysiological targets" that cannot be evaluated with in vitro approaches, allowing a priori the evaluation of a therapeutic response in primary tumors and metastases or in benign diseases.

The evolution of technology, accompanied by improved understanding of so-called molecular imaging, already plays a major role—in combination with pathology—in optimizing a new paradigm, "tailored medicine," in which the focus is primarily on the individual patient rather than the disease.

References

1. Wehner T. The role of functional imaging in the tumor patient. Epilepsia. 2013;54 Suppl 9:44–9.
2. Mansi L, Panza N, Battista C, Pacilio G, Salvatore M. The biological approach to radioimmunoscintigraphy. Biomed Pharmacother. 1990;44(6):295–301.
3. Mansi L. From the magic bullet to an effective therapy: the peptide experience. Eur J Nucl Med Mol Imaging. 2004;31(10):1393–8.
4. Cuccurullo V, Mansi L. Toward tailored medicine (and beyond): the phaeochromocytoma and paraganglioma model. Eur J Nucl Med Mol Imaging. 2012;39(8):1262–5.
5. Westphal SE, Apitzsch J, Penzkofer T, Mahnken AH, Knüchel R. Virtual CT autopsy in clinical pathology: feasibility in clinical autopsies. Virchows Arch. 2012;461(2):211–9.
6. Ayaz H, Onaral B, Izzetoglu K, Shewokis PA, McKendrick R, Parasuraman R. Continuous monitoring of brain dynamics with functional near infrared spectroscopy as a tool for neuroergonomic research: empirical examples and a technological development. Front Hum Neurosci. 2013;7:871.
7. Kircher MF, Willmann JK. Molecular body imaging: MR imaging, CT, and US. Part I. principles. Radiology. 2012;263(3):633–43.
8. Petrella JR. Neuroimaging and the search for a cure for Alzheimer disease. Radiology. 2013;269(3):671–91.
9. Brader P, Wong RJ, Horowitz G, Gil Z. Combination of pet imaging with viral vectors for identification of cancer metastases. Adv Drug Deliv Rev. 2012;64(8):749–55.
10. Mansi L, Virgolini I. Diagnosis and therapy are walking together on radiopeptides' avenue. Eur J Nucl Med Mol Imaging. 2011;38(4):605–12.
11. Grégoire V, Jeraj R, Lee JA, O'Sullivan B. Radiotherapy for head and neck tumours in 2012 and beyond: conformal, tailored, and adaptive? Lancet Oncol. 2012;13(7):e292–300.
12. Kircher MF, Hricak H, Larson SM. Molecular imaging for personalized cancer care. Mol Oncol. 2012;6(2):182–95.
13. Mansi L, Ciarmiello A, Cuccurullo V. PET/MRI and the revolution of the third eye. Eur J Nucl Med Mol Imaging. 2012;39(10):1519–24.

Preclinical Techniques in Animals

8

Francesca Iacobellis, Roberto Grassi, Daniela Berritto, and Luigi Mansi

Introduction

In recent years, new and improved imaging methods have become available, assuming a crucial role in clinical diagnostic evaluation and therapeutic management [1, 2].

This is also reflected in preclinical research, where these methods have shifted the focus of imaging science from anatomical descriptions to the molecular basis of disease [3]. In fact, these new strategies directly integrate cellular and molecular biology concepts and techniques into image generation, enabling comprehensive and noninvasive evaluation of pathophysiological processes in small laboratory animals.

The use of animal models in basic and preclinical research and the opportunity to perform longitudinal studies of the same animal are key factors in the success and timeliness of this approach [4].

Miniaturized versions of clinical diagnostic modalities include, but are not limited to, X-ray, micro-ultrasonography (μUS), micro–magnetic resonance imaging (μMRI), micro–computed tomography (μCT), and radionuclide imaging, including micro–positron emission tomography (μPET) and micro–single photon emission CT (μSPECT). These have all greatly improved our ability to longitudinally study various experimental models of human disease in mice and rodents.

Biomedical imaging techniques for small animals provide one of the most important opportunities for longitudinal research studies to repeatedly examine the same animal model before, during, and after experimental procedures. Noninvasive imaging helps to render animal experiments more ethically acceptable as it is compliant with the principles of the "3Rs" (replacement, reduction, refinement). These principles were formulated in 1959 and encourage researchers to consider "replacing," where possible, the use and/or killing of animals with other equally effective methods; "reducing" the number of experiments; and "refining" techniques to minimize the pain and distress of animals [5, 6]

The aim of this chapter is to describe the most common applications of these techniques and outline their relative advantages and disadvantages. Optical imaging is not considered in this overview because our interest lies in analyzing techniques that are also feasible for diagnostic imaging in humans.

F. Iacobellis (✉) • R. Grassi • D. Berritto • L. Mansi
Sezione Scientifica di Radiodiagnostica, Radioterapia e Medicina Nucleare. Dipartimento Medico Chirurgico di Internistica Clinica e Sperimentale "F. MAGRASSI" e "A. LANZARA", Seconda Università degli Studi di Napoli, Naples, Italy
e-mail: iacobellisf@gmail.com

© Springer Science+Business Media New York 2016
F.M. Sacerdoti et al. (eds.), *Advanced Imaging Techniques in Clinical Pathology*,
Current Clinical Pathology, DOI 10.1007/978-1-4939-3469-0_8

Technique Description

Traditional Radiology (X-Ray)

X-ray examinations provide diagnostically valuable information in a variety of applications. The X-ray instrumentation used for small animal examination (Fig. 8.1) does not differ, in principle, from that in clinical medicine. The main difference lies in the higher resolution levels required, which implies the use of micro-focus X-ray tubes and image detectors with small detector elements [7].

Unenhanced 2D radiographs are typically used to image the skeleton, since the soft tissue contrast is very favorable. Iodinated X-ray contrast media can enhance the contrast of vessels and vascularized areas.

Bone densitometry quantitatively determines bone mineral density (BMD) values via dual-energy X-ray absorptiometry (DXA). It comes under the category of traditional radiology, and the same technique is applied in both animals and in clinical medicine [8–11].

Ultrasound (US)

μUS in animal imaging focuses on investigating accessible biological structures and provides morphological and functional assessment [12]. Based on the propagation of sound waves for imaging soft tissue, μUS is currently available as a dedicated US system for the in vivo imaging of small animals (Fig. 8.2). This device uses much higher frequencies (17–70 MHz) than are used in humans and may produce a resolution below 30 μm. In addition, the use of micro-/nanobubbles with coatings and gas components as a sonographic contrast agent significantly improves sensitivity and enables the measurement of flow in vessels that are 20–30 μm in

Fig. 8.1 Dedicated X-ray instrumentation for small animal examination

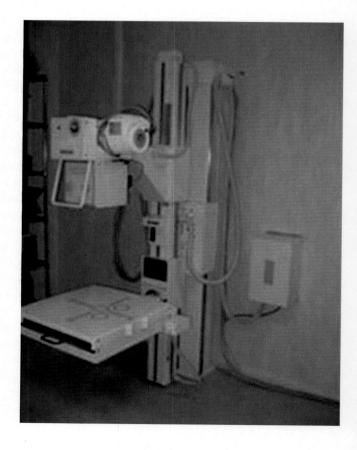

Fig. 8.2 High-resolution
ultrasound instrumentation
for small animal
examination

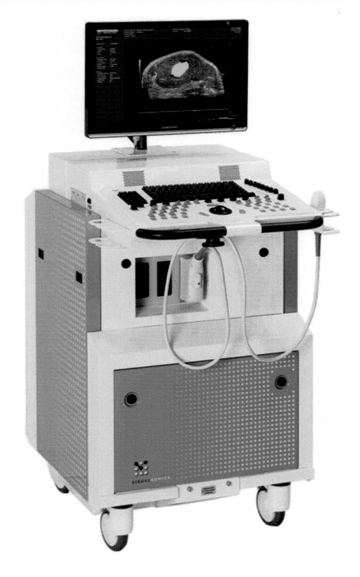

diameter. Ligands or antibodies can also be legated to the coating to make the contrast agent specific and able to selectively bond to certain cell types or processes (e.g., angiogenesis or inflammation) [13, 14]. US is inexpensive, repeatable, fast, noninvasive, readily available and particularly suited to the longitudinal study of small animals. It can be used for noninvasive assessment in abdominal studies [15] or for cardiologic purposes, thanks to the availability of high-frequency ($\geq$40 MHz) transducers and to the ability to record >750 frames per second

using dedicated US systems. As an example, in our experience, echocardiography has been used to monitor the efficacy of gene therapy and/or the progression of dilated cardiomyopathy in BIO 14.6 hamsters. Its value as a tool for repeatable and noninvasive assessment of cardiac diseases in experimental animals has been clearly demonstrated [12].

This technique can also be used to visualize, characterize, and quantify pre-palpable orthotopic and subcutaneous tumors in a multitude of small animal models. Tumors can be

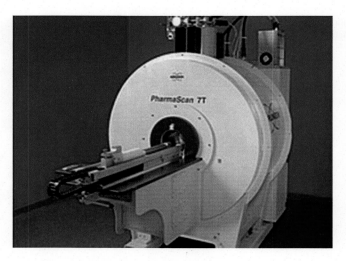

Fig. 8.3 High-resolution magnetic resonance imaging (MRI) instrumentation for small animal examination equipped with several shielded gradients for in vivo applications (<50 μm). This system is also equipped for multinuclear and spectroscopy imaging (i.e., 1H, 31P, 15N,13C, 19F). This instrument includes a breathing and heart gating/monitoring system to limit negative effects on image quality. This feature is essential in the study of animals with high breathing and heart rates

monitored and quantified from tumorigenesis through their growth stages; it is also possible to detect neoplastic involvement of the surrounding tissues and lymph nodes and systemic metastases. Modern software allows the real-time visualization and measurement of tumors in 2D and 3D; blood architecture can be assessed using power and color Doppler and contrast agents for tumor perfusion, also providing informations on neo-angiogenesis [16].

Its real-time nature means μUS could also be useful in guiding drug injection or biopsy and in exploring pregnancy in rats and mice.

Magnetic Resonance Imaging (MRI)

Among the different noninvasive imaging techniques available, μMRI represents a modality of choice because of the high-contrast definition and spatial resolution combined with a high temporal resolution and high safety profile using non-ionizing radiation. MRI provides images of multi-planar sections of the body, examined using magnetic fields and radio waves that act on protons contained within the body [17]. Most small animal imaging with μMRI is performed using horizontal-bore dedicated devices (Fig. 8.3) with a static field ranging from 4.7 to 9.4 T and a 20- to 40-cm tray [18–21]. Systems with even higher static fields, such as 11.7 T and 21.1 T, have also been used [22]. The most commonly used high-field magnets are cryomagnets, in which the low temperatures required for superconductivity are achieved with liquid cooling systems. In our experience, μMRI has been demonstrated as very useful in monitoring intestinal injury in intestinal infarction rat models, providing results comparable with those of pathology [23, 24]. The basic principles of MRI are also applied in spectroscopy, which enables the noninvasive measurement of the levels of some compounds in body tissues [25–28] and in cell tracking where specific contrasts can be used to identify and follow transplanted cells [29, 30]. The resolution of 10–100 μm and the spatial contrast of μMRI systems are not the best among preclinical imaging systems. However, as with other modalities, hybrid systems are being developed, such as MRI/PET, to obtain increasingly complete information from a single device [31–33]. However, MRI alone can already provide functional information using advanced methods, such as those used to evaluate diffusion and perfusion. Thus, the original potential of MRI is optimized, as it can evaluate tissues and lesions with very high diagnostic strength and contrast that does not simply depend on proton density. It can also provide pathophysiological data and is thus more useful in prognosis and therapy.

Computed Tomography (CT)

μCT (Fig. 8.4) is the miniaturization of CT, a technique widely used in clinical diagnostic imaging. Small-animal μCT (mice and rats) can supply very high-resolution anatomical images (up to 9 μm) with 3D views [34]. In daily practice, researchers at some small animal-imaging facilities (SAIFs) tend to limit the study to short scans (around 1 min) to both increase proceeds and reduce radiation exposure, as that can jeopardize longitudinal studies. This technique is balanced by a lower spatial resolution (150–200 μm). μCT systems can be found in many imaging facilities and can cover a variety of applications, with regard to both bone and soft tissue. In terms of the study of bone, a resolution limit of 15 μm should be borne in mind if analyses are to be performed at the trabecular

level. Some μCT systems are able to achieve resolutions that vary from 15 to 90 μm with the same scanner [34]. A device of this kind is clearly very versatile, with a broad range of applications but with the drawback of delivering an elevated dose to the animal at higher resolutions. The optimal resolution for systems dedicated to in vivo studies is 50–100 μm, which allows for a reduced dose and the possibility of longitudinal studies. Specific contrast agents [35] can further improve examination of soft tissue for studies of the heart, angiogenesis, and tumor growth. μCT can also be applied to respiratory diseases. In this case, an additional component is required to control breathing and minimize artifacts caused by the motion of the animal's ribcage. Most systems use a cone-beam X-ray source and a solid-state detector that rotates around the animal, allowing imaging of the entire animal in a single scan. The principal drawbacks of first-generation μCT systems included poor contrast resolution for soft tissue—even after administration of a contrast agent—high radiation doses, long scan times, and image artifacts, particularly at higher resolutions. Second-generation μCT systems incorporated much of the technology used in clinical practice in humans, including arrays with smaller detector

Fig. 8.4 High-resolution computed tomography (CT) instrumentation for small animals (<50 μm). This system uses an X-ray detector with a kV range of 35–80 and an mA range of 0–500. The system has three isotropic resolution settings (27, 45, and 90 μm) with a field of view (FOV) up to 80 mm in diameter. The Locus system uses a CCD with 10-μm square detector element and 100 mm × 50 mm active area. The scan time is 5–60 min depending on the protocol used, with sensitivity in the order of milliMolars

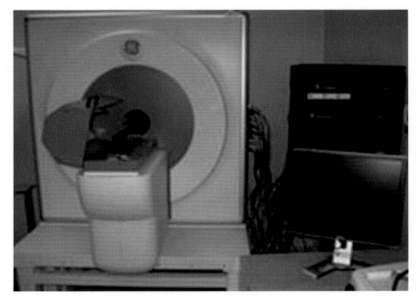

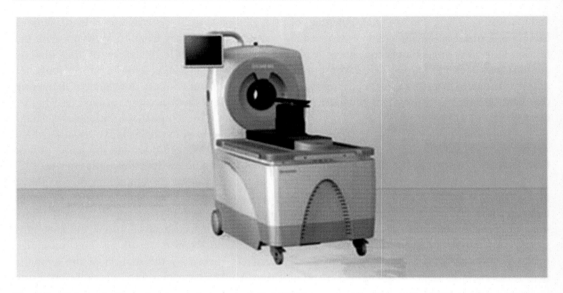

Fig. 8.5 High-resolution positron emission tomography (PET) instrumentation for small animals (spatial resolution of ~1.2 mm in the center of the field, when using OS-EM for image reconstruction)

elements and more powerful X-ray tubes, which enable not only faster scans—0.8 s for the entire animal—but also the use of clinical contrast agents allowing the execution of perfusion studies [36]. In addition, iodinated contrast agents may significantly improve image contrast, enabling the visualization of even small-diameter vessels (20 µm) [37–39]. The major disadvantage of the technique remains the exposure to ionizing radiation, which can alter results of oncologic studies, particularly when repeated follow-up studies are required [37]. µCT systems have traditionally been used to study bone [40–42], thanks to the advantageous contrast between bone and soft tissue. High-resolution µCT systems have also been used with satisfactory results in the study of soft-tissue tumors [43] and in characterizing anatomical phenotypes in transgenic animals [44].

Radionuclide Imaging

Radionuclide imaging techniques, which include µPET (Fig. 8.5) and µSPECT, are functional imaging techniques that detect gamma rays emitted by radiolabeled (positron emitter or gamma emitter) biomolecules introduced into the body so that they accumulate in the tissues of interest. In PET, emission of two high-energy gamma rays (511 kev) are simultaneously detected by two detectors situated 180° apart (an event called coincidence) in the scanner; in SPECT, only one low-energy gamma ray is detected by a single detector [45]. PET is the most selective and sensitive method (in the picomolar to nanomolar range) for widely measuring interactions at the molecular level in vivo [46, 47], and it is being increasingly applied to animal tumor models in several types of studies, from neurological science [48] to preclinical efficacy studies of anticancer agents [49].

As in clinical use in humans, two major advantages of SPECT are the existence of several radiotracers that are based on a variety of radioisotopes with different energies and their relatively longer half-life compared with positron emitters. These properties, together with their wider availability and lower cost, mean they are easily accessible by many research groups. Therefore, those tracers have been well studied and used in not only tumor probing but also in several other biological applications in animal models [48–50].

Hybrid machines have resulted in significant improvements in human and in animal studies. Hybrid machines combining μPET and μCT, or μSPECT and μCT in the same gantry have solved construction issues, allowing the production of hybrid PET-MRI systems permitting the simultaneous acquisition of the two images [51–53]. Furthermore, high-performing machines integrating a PET scanner with a 9.4 T MR scanner have been produced [54].

References

1. Grassi R, Lagalla R, Rotondo A. Genomics, proteomics, MEMS and SAIF: which role for diagnostic imaging? Radiol Med. 2008;113(6):775–8.
2. Yang X. Interventional molecular imaging. Radiology. 2010;254(3):651–4.
3. Blasberg R, Piwnica-Worms D. Imaging: strategies, controversies, and opportunities. Clin Cancer Res. 2012;18(3):631–7.
4. Grassi R, Cavaliere C, Cozzolino S, Mansi L, Cirillo S, Tedeschi G, Franchi R, Russo P, Cornacchia S, Rotondo A. Small animal imaging facility: new perspectives for the radiologist. Radiol Med. 2009;114(1):152–67.
5. Russell WM, Burch RL. The principles of humane experimental technique. In: Russell WM, Burch RL, editors. The progress of humane technique. Springfield IL: Charles C. Thomas; 1959.
6. Flecknell P. Replacement, reduction and refinement. ALTEX. 2002;19(2):73as.
7. Kalender WA, Deak P, Engelke K, Karolczak M. X-Ray and X-Ray-CT. In: Kiressing F, Pichler BJ, editors. Small animal imaging. Berlin: Springer-Verlag; 2011. p. 125–39.
8. Kastl S, Sommer T, Klein W, Hohenberger W, Engelke K. Accuracy and precision of bone mineral density and bone mineral content in excised rat humeri using fan beam dual energy X-ray absorptiometry. Bone. 2002;30(1):243–6.
9. Libouban H, Simon Y, Silve C, et al. Comparison of pencil-, fan-, and cone-beam dual X mineral density and bone mineral content in excised rat humeri using fan beam dual ener. Densitom. 2002;5(4):355–61.
10. Soon G, Quintin A. Scalfo F et al PIXImus bone densitometer and associated technical measurement issues of skeletal growth in the young rat. Calcif Tissue Int. 2006;78(3):186–92.
11. Nazarian A, Cory E, Muller R, Snyder BD. Shortcomings of DXA to assess changes in bone tissue density and microstructure induced by

metabolic bone diseases in rat models. Osteoporos Int. 2009;20(1):123–32.
12. Belfiore MP, Berritto D, Iacobellis F, Rossi C, Nigro G, Rotundo IL, Cozzolino S, Cappabianca S, Rotondo A, Grassi R. A longitudinal study on BIO14.6 hamsters with dilated cardiomyopathy: micro-echocardiographic evaluation. Cardiovasc Ultrasound. 2011;9:39.
13. Lanza GM, Wickline SA. Targeted ultrasonic contrast agents for molecular imaging and therapy. Prog Cardiovasc Dis. 2001;44(4):132001.
14. Dayton PA, Ferrara KW. Targeted imaging using ultrasound. J Magn Reson Imaging. 2002;16 (4):3622002.
15. Iacobellis F, Berritto D, Belfiore MP, Di Lanno I, Maiorino M, Saba L, Grassi R. Meaning of free intraperitoneal fluid in small-bowel obstruction: preliminary results using high-frequency microsonography in a rat model. J Ultrasound Med. 2014;33(5):887–93.
16. Foster S and Theodoropoulos C. Ultrasound. In Kiressing F, Pichler BJ, Small animal imaging. 2011 Springer-Verlag Berlin Heidelberg pp.207-217.
17. Jakob P. Small animal magnetic resonance imaging: basic principles, instrumentation and practical issue. In: Kiressing F, Pichler BJ, editors. Small animal imaging. Berlin: Springer-Verlag; 2011. p. 151–64.
18. Berritto D, Iacobellis F, Belfiore MP, Rossi C, Saba L, Grassi R. Early MRI findings of small bowel obstruction: an experimental study in rats. Radiol Med. 2014;119(6):377–83.
19. Somma F, Berritto D, Iacobellis F, Landi N, Cavaliere C, Corona M, Russo S, Di Mizio R, Rotondo A, Grassi R. 7T an experimental study in rats. Radiol rat model: timing of the appearance of findings. Magn Reson Imaging. 2013;31(3):408–13.
20. Berritto D, Iacobellis F, Somma F, Corona M, Faggian A, Iacomino A, Feragalli B, Saba L, La Porta M, Grassi R. 7T mMR in the assessment of acute arterial mesenteric ischemia in a rat model. J Biol Regul Homeost Agents. 2013;27(3):771–9.
21. Saba L, Berritto D, Iacobellis F, Scaglione M, Castaldo S, Cozzolino S, Mazzei MA, Di Mizio V, Grassi R. Acute arterial mesenteric ischemia and reperfusion: macroscopic and MRI findings, preliminary report. World J Gastroenterol. 2013;19 (40):6825–33.
22. Beck B, Plant DH, Grant SC, Thelwall PE, Silver X, Mareci TH, Benveniste H, Smith M, Collins C, Crozier S, Blackband SJ. Progress in high field MRI at the University of Florida. MAGMA. 2002;13 (3):152–7.
23. Iacobellis F, Berritto D, Somma F, Cavaliere C, Corona M, Cozzolino S, Fulciniti F, Cappabianca S, Rotondo A, Grassi R. Magnetic resonance imaging: a new tool for diagnosis of acute ischemic colitis? World J Gastroenterol. 2012;18(13):1496–501.

24. Berritto D, Somma F, Landi N, Cavaliere C, Corona M, Russo S, Fulciniti F, Cappabianca S, Rotondo A, Grassi R. Seven-Tesla micro-MRI in early detection of acute arterial ischaemia: evolution of findings in an in vivo rat model. Radiol Med. 2011;116(6):829–41.

25. Kauppinen RA, Peet AC. Using magnetic resonance imaging and spectroscopy in cancer diagnostics and monitoring: preclinical and clinical approaches. Cancer Biol Ther. 2011;12(8):665–79.

26. Borges AR, Lopez-Larrubia P, Marques JB, Cerdan SG. MR imaging features of high-grade gliomas in murine models: how they compare with human disease, reflect tumor biology, and play a role in preclinical trials. AJNR Am J Neuroradiol. 2012;33 (1):24–36.

27. Zhu H, Barker PB. MR spectroscopy and spectroscopic imaging of the brain. Methods Mol Biol. 2011;711:203–26.

28. Kurhanewicz J, Bok R, Nelson SJ, Vigneron DB. Current and potential applications of clinical 13C MR spectroscopy. J Nucl Med. 2008;49 (3):341–4.

29. Modo M. Tracking transplanted cells by MRI—methods and protocols. Methods Mol Biol. 2011;771:717–32.

30. Weissleder R, Moore A, Mahmood U, Bhorade R, Benveniste H, Chiocca EA, Basilion JP. In vivo magnetic resonance imaging of transgene expression. Nat Med. 2000;6(3):351–5.

31. Slates RB, Farahani K, Shao Y, Marsden PK, Taylor J, Summers PE, Williams S, Beech J, Cherry SR. A study of artifacts in simultaneous PET and MR imaging using a prototype MR compatible PET scanner. Phys Med Biol. 1999;44(8):2015–27.

32. Faccioli N, Marzola P, Boschi F, Sbarbati A, D'Onofrio M, Pozzi MR. Pathological animal models in the experimental evaluation of tumour microvasculature with magnetic resonance imaging. Radiol Med. 2007;112(3):319–28.

33. Menon RS, Kim SG. Spatial and temporal limits in cognitive neuroimaging with fMRI. Trends Cogn Sci. 1999;3(6):207–16.

34. Ritman EL. Molecular imaging in small animals-roles for micro-CT. J Cell Biochem. 2002;39:116–24.

35. Goertzen AL, Meadors AK, Silverman RW, Cherry SR. Simultaneous molecular and anatomical imaging of the mouse in vivo. Phys Med Biol. 2002;47 (24):4315–28.

36. Suckow C, Stout D. Micro CT liver contrast agent enhancement over time, dose, and mouse strain. Mol Imaging Biol. 2008;10(2):114–20.

37. Savai R, Wolf JC, Greschus S, Eul BG, Schermuly RT, Hänze J, Voswinckel R, Langheinrich AC, Grimminger F, Traupe H, Seeger W, Rose F. Analysis of tumor vessel supply in Lewis lung carcinoma in mice by fluorescent microsphere distribution and imaging with micro- and flat-panel

computed tomography. Am J Pathol. 2005;167 (4):937–46.

38. Marxen M, Thornton MM, Chiarot CB, Klement G, Koprivnikar J, Sled JG, Henkelman RM. Micro CT scanner performance and considerations for vascular specimen imaging. Med Phys. 2004;31(2):305–13.

39. Bhattacharjee D, Ito A. Deceleration of carcinogenic potential by adaptation with low dose gamma irradiation. In Vivo. 2001;15:87–92.

40. Borah B, Gross GJ, Dufresne TE, Smith TS, Cockman MD, Chmielewski PA, Lundy MW, Hartke JR, Sod EW. Three-dimensional microimaging (MRmicroI and microCT), finite element modeling, and rapid prototyping provide unique insights into bone architecture in osteoporosis. Anat Rec. 2001;265 (2):101–10.

41. Van Rietbergen B, Majumdar S, Pistoia W, Newitt DC, Kothari M, Laib A, Rietbergen B, Majumdar S. Pistoiellous bone mechanical properties from micro-FE models based on micro-CT, pQCT and MR images. Technol Health Care. 1998;6 (5-6):413–20.

42. Ruegsegger P, Koller B, Muller R. A micro tomographic system for the non-destructive evaluation of bone architecture. Calcif Tissue Int. 1996;58:24–9.

43. Kennel SJ, Davis IA, Branning J, Pan H, Kabalka GW, Paulus MJ. High resolution computed tomography and MRI for monitoring lung tumor growth in mice undergoing radioimmunotherapy: correlation with histology. Med Phys. 2000;27(5):1101–7.

44. Paulus MJ, Gleason SS, Sari-Sarraf H, et al. High-resolution X-ray CT screening of mutant mouse models. Proc SPIE. 2000;3921:270.

45. Ray P. Multimodality molecular imaging of disease progression in living subjects. J Biosci. 2011;36:499–504.

46. Jones T. The role of positron emission tomography within the spectrum of medical imaging. Eur J Nucl Med. 1996;23:207–11.

47. Lammertsma AA. Role of human and animal PET studies in drug development Int. Congr. Ser., 1265 (2004), pp. 3(19).

48. Xi W, Tian M, Zhang H. Molecular imaging in neuroscience research with small-animal PET in rodents. Neurosci Res. 2011;70(2):133–43.

49. Toyohara J, Ishiwata K. Animal tumor models for PET in drug development. Ann Nucl Med. 2011;25:717–31.

50. Meikle SR, Kench P, Kassiou M, Banati RB. Small animal SPECT and its place in the matrix of molecular imaging technologies. Phys Med Biol. 2005;50(22): R45–61.

51. Herzog H, Van Den Hoff J. Combined PET/MR systems: an overview and comparison of currently available options. Q J Nucl Med Mol Imaging. 2012;56(3):247–67.

52. Wagenaar DJ, Kapusta M, Li J, Patt BE. Rationale for the combination of nuclear medicine with magnetic

resonance for pre-clinical imaging. Technol Cancer Res Treat. 2006;5(4):343–50.

53. Tatsumi M, Yamamoto S, Imaizumi M, Watabe T, Kanai Y, Aoki M, Kato H, Shimosegawa E, Hatazawa J. Simultaneous PET/MR body imaging in rats: initial experiences with an integrated PET/MRI scanner. Ann Nucl Med. 2012;23 [Epub ahead of print].

54. Maramraju SH, Smith SD, Junnarkar SS, Schulz D, Stoll S, Ravindranath B, Purschke ML, Rescia S, Southekal S, Pratte JF, Vaska P, Woody CL, Schlyer DJ. Small animal simultaneous PET/MRI: initial experiences in a 9.4 T MicroMRI. Phys Med Biol. 2011;56(8):2459–80. Epub 2011 Mar 25.

Preclinical Imaging: Experimental Example 9

Daniela Berritto, Roberto Grassi, Francesca Iacobellis,
Claudia Rossi, and Luigi Mansi

Introduction

This chapter is an addendum to the previous one, which briefly described the most important diagnostic imaging techniques used in preclinical animal imaging and their possible relationship with pathology. In particular, we report an example from our own experience; we present the abilities of micro–magnetic resonance imaging (μMRI) in biomedical research evaluating animal models of complex pathological human diseases.

After defining the scope, we start with a general premise describing μMRI as an imaging modality that can dynamically explore the mechanisms of disease in vivo. This goal is reached by collecting anatomical, functional, and metabolic informations noninvasively and, when possible, almost simultaneously.

The example we present regards the characterization of bowel ischemic disease. The role of μMRI can be seen from the images expressing different features as an expression of different pathophysiological mechanisms.

The lesson learned is that μMRI and, more generally, animal imaging, may help pathologists studying pathophysiological premises that determine pathological findings. This may be achieved using available machines that allow functional studies at a spatial resolution of up to microns. The chapter concludes with an updated bibliography.

Scope

Because this chapter is an addendum to the previous one, which described technological tools for preclinical animal imaging, we want to highlight the use of μMRI as a helpful support to the pathophysiological comprehension of lesions observed by a pathologist. To this end, we refer to an example from our own experience of characterizing bowel ischemic disease via μMRI.

Magnetic Resonance for Animal Imaging (μMRI)

In biomedical research, many experimental studies require the application of small animal models for complex human diseases, where the underlying disease mechanisms can be explored in vivo by collecting—noninvasively and, when possible, simultaneously—anatomical, functional, and metabolic information [1–3]. Therefore,

D. Berritto (✉) • R. Grassi • F. Iacobellis • C. Rossi •
L. Mansi
Sezione Scientifica di Radiodiagnostica, Radioterapia
e Medicina Nucleare. Dipartimento Medico Chirurgico di
Internistica Clinica e Sperimentale "F. MAGRASSI"
e "A. LANZARA", Seconda Università degli Studi di
Napoli, Naples, Italy
e-mail: berritto.daniela@gmail.com

© Springer Science+Business Media New York 2016
F.M. Sacerdoti et al. (eds.), *Advanced Imaging Techniques in Clinical Pathology*,
Current Clinical Pathology, DOI 10.1007/978-1-4939-3469-0_9

demand is strong in animal research for imaging modalities that can provide these informations in vivo, in longitudinal studies, using 3D techniques without limits determined by depth resolution, as in optical imaging. Among the currently available noninvasive imaging techniques, magnetic resonance imaging (MRI) is frequently a first choice as it has a number of favorable characteristics that make it an ideal candidate for a broad range of imaging tasks: extraordinary 3D representation capabilities; high spatial resolution; excellent contrast abilities, and possible functional and molecular analyses, including those without contrast media. All these favorable features are combined with a high safety profile as no harmful ionizing radiation is applied.

Therefore, the role of MRI is ever increasing, not only in medical imaging, where it occupies a primary position in the diagnostic tree for a large series of diseases, but also in biomedical research.

When MRI is constructed as a tool for small animal imaging μMRI, it is substantially based on the same physical principles as its clinical counterpart, MRI. Conversely, μMRI scanners are many times more powerful, being produced using the best performing and most expensive materials. Furthermore, they have a more effective geometry, are constrained by less stringent ethical and technical contraindications, and are able to use 9.4T scanners, which are not yet available for use in humans, where the technological frontier does not exceed 3T.

Given the power of these machines, μMRI is now being increasingly exploited to provide informations in animal models, focusing on revealing anatomical and physiological changes during disease progression or in response to potential therapeutic treatment.

Image sets can be obtained with a resolution of 30–100 μm in all dimensions, in living animals, with the possibility of visualizing images of the whole animal or specific organs, represented in arbitrary planes.

This extended capability of μMRI requires more advanced machinery able to reach a tenfold increase in spatial resolution in all three dimensions. To overcome this barrier, the development of specific μMRI technology was necessary, with more powerful magnets, dedicated receiver coils and chains, stronger gradient sets, new image acquisition sequences, and, finally, biological support for small animals in a high magnetic field [4].

In general, μMRI requires the small animals to be immobilized and thus anesthetized. Inhaled anesthetics such as isoflurane, or intravenous anesthetics such as propofol, are commonly used and are administered via a nose cone or tail vein catheter and allow for short induction and recovery times. While under anesthesia, the temperature of the animal must be kept constant at 37 °C using either warm airflow and circulating water or electrical pads, since the temperature inside the magnet core ranges from 15 to 20 °C. In general, the vital functions of the animals during anesthesia must be carefully controlled.

Characterization of Bowel Ischemic Disease via μMRI

Gastrointestinal tract ischemia and infarction constitute different clinical syndromes characterized by inadequate blood perfusion to the bowel and represent a life-threatening vascular emergency with high mortality [5–7]. Early diagnosis is the key to reducing the death rate and to improving quality of life.

Diagnostic imaging of bowel ischemic disease reflects the complexity of the pathophysiological mechanisms [8–12].

The ability to reproduce human diseases in animal models enables us to increase our knowledge of the physiopathology of these disorders and also enables the study of new diagnostic and therapeutic approaches [13–16].

Different etiological varieties of bowel ischemic diseases exist, and a rat model of each type may be designed (respectively, by ligation of superior and/or inferior mesenteric artery and superior mesenteric vein) to exactly define the onset and the development of the lesions, as well

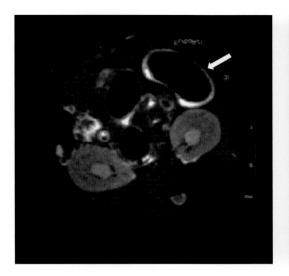 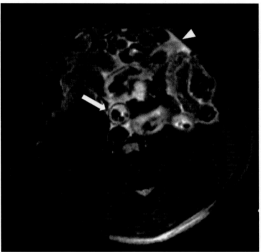

Fig. 9.1 Axial T2-weighted micro–magnetic resonance image (μMRI) of the rat's bowel depicting wall hyperintensity (*arrow*)

Fig. 9.2 Axial T2-weighted micro–magnetic resonance image (μMRI) of the rat's bowel: presence of free fluid in the abdominal cavity (*arrowhead*); bowel loop dilation with gas–fluid luminal content (*arrow*)

as to compare histological and macroscopic features with μMRI findings.

In animal models of acute bowel ischemia/infarction, μMRI offered the major advantage of noninvasively obtaining detailed anatomical and physiological informations in one imaging session. These data, obtained using a longitudinal approach, could be exploited for a significantly improved characterization of this pathology.

The ischemic/μMRI protocol used a 7 T system.

Figure 9.1 shows an axial T2-weighted μMRI image of the rat's bowel depicting wall hyperintensity which represents one of the earliest and most common findings of bowel ischemia/infarction [12–14]. The bowel wall hyperintensity was clarified by histological analysis, which demonstrated the presence of subepithelial (Grunhagen's) space, due to the development of edema.

The following parameters were also assessed using μMRI: presence of free fluid and/or gas in the abdominal cavity; diameter of bowel loops and luminal content (gas and/or fluid); mucosal thickness; mesenteric engorgement; and wall pneumatosis (Fig. 9.2). Magnetic resonance angiography is another powerful tool that can be realized in vivo via μMRI to image blood vessels. These images, unlike conventional or computed tomography (CT) angiography, do not display the lumen of the vessel, but rather the blood flowing through the vessel without using contrast media.

In our experiments, FLASH TOF 2D sequences were performed and subsequently reconstructed with maximum intensity projection (MIP) images to demonstrate the correct vascular ligation and the lack of flow after surgery.

In summary, this imaging example was chosen to demonstrate the plethora of information available with μMRI that can be exploited for improved tissue characterization in animal models.

Compared with histological analysis and macroscopic evidence, the μMRI succeeded in identifying the early signs of ischemia/infarction just 1 h after vascular occlusion.

Furthermore, our study provided a chronological progression of the radiological findings related to macroscopic and histological features; this is the prerequisite to obtaining an early diagnosis and providing treatment, thereby determining a better prognosis for the patient.

Lessons Learned

In this chapter, we have demonstrated, with an example from our own experience, how preclinical imaging may help the pathologist. In particular, we were able to study pathophysiological premises determining pathological findings. This goal may be reached experimentally in animal models because of the high performance of available machines, allowing spatial resolution up to microns.

In this sense, animal imaging may represent a major improvement in research, mainly when functional techniques are available. In fact, repeatable acquisitions in living beings are possible, enabling the acquisition of a series of relevant information that pathology alone cannot achieve.

References

1. Grassi R, Lagalla R, Rotondo A. Genomics, proteomics, MEMS and SAIF: which role for diagnostic imaging? Radiol Med. 2008;113:775–8.
2. Grassi R, Cavaliere C, Cozzolino S, Mansi L, Cirillo S, Tedeschi G, Franchi R, Russo P, Cornacchia S, Rotondo A. Small animal imaging facility: new perspectives for the radiologist. Radiol Med. 2009;114:152–67.
3. Belfiore MP, Berritto D, Iacobellis F, Rossi C, Nigro G, Rotondo IL, Cozzolino S, Cappabianca S, Rotondo A, Grassi R. A longitudinal study on BIO14.6 hamsters with dilated cardiomyopathy: micro-echocardiographic evaluation. Cardiovasc Ultrasound. 2011;9.
4. Peter Jakob. Small Animal Magnetic Resonance Imaging: Basic Principles, Instrumentation and Practical Issue 2011, Part 3, 151–164.
5. Gore RM, Yaghmai V, Thakrar KH, Berlin JW, Newmark GM, Mehta UK, Miller FH. Imaging in intestinal ischemic disorders. Radiol Clin North Am. 2008;46(5):845–75.
6. Paterno F, Longo WE. The etiology and pathogenesis of vascular disorders of the intestine. Radiol Clin North Am. 2008;46(5):877–85. v.
7. Reginelli A, Mandato Y, Solazzo A, Berritto D, Iacobellis F, Grassi R. Errors in the radiological evaluation of the alimentary tract: part II. Semin Ultrasound CT MR. 2012;33(4):308–17.
8. Angelelli G, Scardapane A, Memeo M, Stabile Ianora AA, Rotondo A. Acute bowel ischemia: CT findings. Eur J Radiol. 2004;50:37–47.
9. Schoots IG, Koffeman GI, Legemate DA, Levi M, van Gulik TM. Systematic review of survival after acute mesenteric ischaemia according to disease aetiology. Br J Surg. 2004;91:17–27.
10. Oldenburg WA, Lau LL, Rodenberg TJ, Edmonds HJ, Burger CD. Acute mesenteric ischemia: a clinical review. Arch Intern Med. 2004;164:1054–62.
11. Sreenarasimhaiah J. Diagnosis and management of intestinal ischaemic disorders. BMJ. 2003;326:1372–6.
12. Romano S, Romano L, Grassi R. Multidetector row computed tomography findings from ischemia to infarction of the large bowel. Eur J Radiol. 2007;61(3):433–41.
13. Mazzei MA, Mazzei FG, Marrelli D, Imbriaco G, Guerrini S, Vindigni C, Civitelli S, Roviello F, Grassi R, Volterrani L. Computed tomographic evaluation of mesentery: diagnostic value in acute mesenteric ischemia. J Comput Assist Tomogr. 2012;36(1):1–7.
14. Iacobellis F, Berritto D, Somma F, Cavaliere C, Corona M, Cozzolino S, Fulciniti F, Cappabianca S, Rotondo A. Grassi R Magnetic resonance imaging: a new tool for diagnosis of acute ischemic colitis? World J Gastroenterol. 2012;18(13):1496–501.
15. Berritto D, Somma F, Landi N, Cavaliere C, Corona M, Russo S, Fulciniti F, Cappabianca S, Rotondo A, Grassi R. Seven-Tesla micro-MRI in early detection of acute arterial ischaemia: evolution of findings in an in vivo rat model. Radiol Med. 2011;116:829–41.
16. Somma F, Berritto D, Iacobellis F, Landi N, Cavaliere C, Corona M, Russo S, Di Mizio R, Rotondo A, Grassi R. 7T µMRI of mesenteric venous ischemia in a rat model: timing of the appearance of findings Magnetic Resonance Imaging 2012.

Clinical Techniques in Humans

10

Luigi Mansi, Vincenzo Cuccurullo, and Roberto Grassi

Scope

We briefly describe the main characteristics, advantages, and limitations of the most widely available diagnostic imaging (DI) techniques.

Traditional Radiology

Traditional radiology includes all planar examinations performed using X-rays. As the image is based on differences in density, the best results are achieved where a favorable lesion-to-background ratio is easily reached, as in the lungs and breast, where lesions present early with a higher opacity than the surrounding normal tissue. Thus, detection of millimetric (and occasionally submillimetric) lesions is possible. Similarly, satisfactory results are possible at the skeletal level, where pathological alterations may determine changes in opacity compared with healthy bone. In particular, the administration of contrast media can artificially increase (or, less frequently, decrease) normal contrast, thereby enabling the analysis of vessels,

ureters, gastrointestinal lumen, and some parenchyma, which would otherwise be impossible with a standard approach.

Standard techniques, such as chest or skeletal X-ray, are fast, cheap, easily performed, and available everywhere, even at the bedside. They can be a first-line diagnostic tool in cases where satisfactory diagnostic accuracy is possible, for instance, in a limited number of cases such as skeletal fractures and suspicious pulmonary lesions. Limits relate to the radiation dose, the lower accuracy than alternative techniques, the limited context of analysis, and ineffectiveness in evaluating many cases, such as those involving lymph nodes, brain, liver metastases, and the mediastinum [1].

Dedicated examinations, such as mammography (Mx), are performed with a specific system and using a particular methodology. Mx remains the best first-line approach for the screening and diagnosis of breast cancer, primarily in postmenopausal women. It is cost effective compared with ultrasound (US) and magnetic resonance imaging (MRI), despite using ionizing radiation. Nevertheless, when results are positive, further insights may be required to increase diagnostic accuracy, as Mx is less effective in dense breast tissue (as is the case in some young subjects, in the presence of prostheses, and in detecting recurrence after radiotherapy) [2–4].

Radiological studies use contrast media to enhance the contrast of structures or fluids

L. Mansi (✉) • V. Cuccurullo • R. Grassi
Sezione Scientifica di Radiodiagnostica, Radioterapia e Medicina Nucleare. Dipartimento Medico Chirurgico di Internistica Clinica e Sperimentale "F. MAGRASSI" e "A. LANZARA", Seconda Università degli Studi di Napoli, Naples, Italy
e-mail: luigi.mansi@unina2.it

© Springer Science+Business Media New York 2016
F.M. Sacerdoti et al. (eds.), *Advanced Imaging Techniques in Clinical Pathology*,
Current Clinical Pathology, DOI 10.1007/978-1-4939-3469-0_10

within the body [5]. Currently, the most commonly used are those that enhance the visibility of blood vessels (iodinated agents used in angiography) and of the gastrointestinal tract (barium). Less widely used are functional studies as pyeloureterography. Radiological techniques with contrast media are disadvantaged by requiring a high radiation charge and by side effects, which are sometimes absolute contraindications; preserved renal function is also essential. These days, angiographic techniques are used primarily as a second-line diagnostic step, preferably before and/or during therapeutic revascularization procedures. The clinical role of barium studies is currently more limited compared with invasive methods that allow biopsy; their role has been further decreased with the advent of tridimensional fast computed tomography (CT) scans that can also provide information on the gastrointestinal lumen [6].

Computed Tomography (CT)

CT is currently the major radiological technique used, with X-rays allowing 3D spatial and structural analysis based on differences in density [7]; CT can also be used to evaluate structures that are invisible with traditional radiotherapy, such as the mediastinum and soft tissues. The introduction of spiral CT signifies a significant technological improvement that enables rapid volumetric analysis and has led to new technical achievements, such as coronary CT [8]. Contrast media can also be used with CT, which is very helpful because it can not only provide angiographic information but also contribute to a differential diagnosis with parenchymal lesions. Whereas the high radiation dose [9] (although this has decreased significantly with recent technologies) and side effects can render it an absolute contraindication, CT represents a first-line tool in DI for many indications, with a primary role in both oncology (diagnosis, staging, re-staging) and non-oncology indications, such as in emergency medicine [10].

Ultrasound (US)

Ultrasonography is a technique based on US and is therefore performed without ionizing radiation. As such, it represents a safe first-line procedure in DI and is now almost mandatory in pregnancy and is a priori cost effective in pediatrics [11]. US is relatively inexpensive compared with CT and MRI and is widely available, including at the bedside and in emergencies. Its value is increased by its high diagnostic accuracy when used to evaluate both superficial and deep structures such as skin, muscles, joints, soft tissues, thyroid, liver, breast, and lymph nodes, while also useful in the diagnosis of renal and biliary colic and to guide biopsy and/or therapeutic procedures. The basic information it provides mainly discriminates between solid and liquid components, defined in a wide range of structural variations and distinct morphologically, with limitations in defining calcifications and gaseous components. Sonography may be implemented with Doppler measurements, and contrast media adds further data mainly to do with vascularity and permeability. Doppler techniques also enable the analysis of vessels and echocardiography, now first-line procedures in cardiovascular diseases [12]. Diagnostic performance may be increased using endo-vaginal, endo-rectal, and transesophageal transducers, leading US to take a primary role as an intra-surgical technique. However, US also has limitations. First, US is unable to penetrate bone and performs very poorly in the presence of gas. Therefore, CT is of no use in evaluating skeletal diseases or organs covered by bone, such as the adult brain. Furthermore, it can provide no information on lungs, and analysis of the gastrointestinal tract can be very difficult. Further difficulties can be encountered in obese subjects, mainly in the evaluation of deep structures, or in echocardiography, where technical problems occur with the acoustic window in patients with emphysema or with malformation of the chest. Operator dependency is a major problem: differences in reproducibility have been found between sonographers or at follow-up studies with the same operator, mainly using different machines. This is a disadvantage because ultrasonography is not panoramic and can thus favor false-negative results, mainly for inexperienced sonographers, as frequently found in programs where many different operators screen large populations. Finally, US can provide a final diagnosis in only a limited number of conditions, and therefore further insights are frequently required [13].

Magnetic Resonance (MR)

MRI is based on the magnetic properties of some typical nuclei of atoms. First of all is hydrogen; however, it is also possible to analyze other nuclei such as helium-3, lithium-7, fluorine-19, oxygen-17, sodium-23, phosphorus-31, and xenon-129 with higher-performance MR scanners and primarily in research situations. This advanced analysis could be an interesting clinical tool in the future that may enable the imaging of organs usually poorly visualized at 1H MRI (e.g., lungs and bones) as well as promising wider metabolic and functional evaluations [14].

Starting with the capability to define proton density, MRI can produce multiparametric images depending on the molecular context. Different tissue variables, including spin density, T1 and T2 relaxation times, flow, and spectral shifts, can be used to construct images. It is possible to define the best contrast for each body compartment and in relation to the specific clinical problem, as well as adding information on the molecular environment [14, 15]. Further improvement, both increasing contrast and adding functional and biochemical data, is possible with advanced MR techniques such as functional MRI (fMRI), diffusion MRI, or MR spectroscopy (MRS). Thus, evidence of altered function or of a molecular event preceding pathological changes can be observed; this will enable earlier and more accurate diagnosis as well as provide prognostic information. In particular, high contrast may be acquired in soft tissue without significant difference in atomic density. Therefore, MRI has advantages over

CT in many pathological conditions because of the better lesion-to-background ratio that is possible in, for example, demyelinating cerebral diseases and/or in evaluating lesions in territories such as the pelvis, head, or neck. Conversely CT, which sometimes has problems evidencing or correctly locating minimal structural changes, has technical primacy over MRI when evaluating bone and lungs or detecting calcification, i.e., in molecular structures with low 1H content. A further significant advantage of CT is its speed, which enables studies in pediatrics and psychiatric patients without necessarily requiring narcosis or sedation, which is often required with MRI.

MRI has an advantage over CT and nuclear medicine as it does not use ionizing radiation, a favorable situation for pregnant and pediatric patients. Nevertheless, MRI is a costly and complex method that is also slower and less widely available than CT and therefore not as cost effective as CT. CT therefore remains favored in many comparative situations; in particular, there are currently no significant indications for MRI in emergency medicine. Furthermore, although MRI does not use ionizing radiation, it does have contraindications, being unfeasible in many patients such as those with metal implants or pacemakers. MRI also carries risks for patients after intravenous administration of contrast media, which can result in a life-threatening renal syndrome. The most widely used MRI contrast media are paramagnetic substances containing gadolinium, which, when administered intravenous, can enhance the appearance of blood vessels, tumors, or inflammation, through information mainly to do with vascularity and permeability. Contrast agents may also be administered orally or directly injected, such as into a joint in the case of arthrograms. The newest contrast agents, including paramagnetic substances with manganese or super-paramagnetic iron agents, may further increase diagnostic accuracy, such as in the detection of liver metastases. As MRI performed with a standard scanner is a time-consuming procedure requiring the patient to lie supine within an oppressive gantry, subjects with claustrophobia are contraindicated; however, this problem has been surpassed with the use of "open scanners", although they are not as good. Conversely, while high-performance MR machines such as 3 T scanners are now available in clinical practice, they are not widespread. The most powerful systems, capable of very high spatial and contrast resolution and able to distinguish between two arbitrarily similar but not identical tissues, remain most in use in preclinical animal research [15].

The value of MRI lies in the ability to define the best imaging condition for each clinical problem, utilizing a complex library of pulse sequences, each of which is optimized to provide a particular image contrast. Conversely, this advantage creates operator dependence in the choice of the best technique, reliant on the competence of the individual physician and technologist involved in the scan.

Whereas T1- and T2-weighted MRI are the clinical "workhorses," multiparametric imaging can benefit from other basic and specialized MR scans. Diffusion MRI is particularly relevant because it can measure the diffusion of water molecules in biological tissues. Diffusion tensor imaging (DTI) [15] and diffusion-weighted imaging (DWI) can, with further information when coupled with imaging of cerebral perfusion, provide very relevant diagnostic information, and can also obtain data useful for a prognostic framework and to better define a therapeutic strategy. An anatomic pattern substantially overlapped with that obtained with invasive angiographic techniques enables MR angiography, with or without contrast media, to correctly detect stenosis and aneurysms.

MRS also contributes important information, although it has a lower spatial resolution and is only able to evaluate a restricted field of view. It measures the levels of different metabolites in body tissues but requires higher field strengths (3 T and above); MRS can provide biochemical information regarding molecules containing not only 1H but also other elements such as 31P, making a helpful contribution to improved metabolic analysis.

More recently, two of the major limitations of MRI have been overcome. First, it became possible to use MRI as a guide in interventional procedures using non-ferromagnetic instruments in open MR scanners. Similarly, technological evolution saw the construction of hybrid positron emission tomography (PET)–MRI systems with a single gantry, utilizing a PET scanner not affected by the magnetic field.

Nuclear Medicine

Nuclear medicine is a medical specialty that uses radionuclides for diagnosis and therapy. Whereas radioisotopes emitting (directly or indirectly) low doses of electromagnetic radiation (i.e., gamma rays or positrons) are used for diagnosis, radionuclide therapy is based on the administration of high doses of corpuscular nuclear (beta minus and alpha) radiation with the intention of obtaining a deterministic therapeutic effect. Within the scope of this book, we discuss only diagnostic nuclear medicine, if not otherwise specifically reported.

In terms of machines detecting gamma radiation, we first have laboratory detectors, called gamma or beta counters, which are primarily used to measure radioactivity in biological samples but are also used to evaluate radioactive contamination.

Next are probes that measure radioactivity in vivo in humans without producing images. Within this group, there is a lot of interest in probes used for so-called radio-guided surgery (RGS), which is very helpful in guiding the surgeon to the goal (such as in the detection of the sentinel lymph node in breast cancer).

The standard imaging machine in nuclear medicine is the gamma camera, which can produce static or dynamic scintigraphies. The tomographic systems, which enable tridimensional analysis, are distinct in single photon emission CT (SPECT), when using gamma emitters, and PET, where the signal originates from radionuclides emitting positrons.

The computer plays a central role in nuclear medicine; it is needed not only for technical issues such as tomographic reconstructions but also for reliable quantitative analysis. It is also possible to detect non-focal diseases, better analyze changes at follow-up or post-therapy, acquire implemental data for a differential diagnosis, and more rigorously define stress tests. Importantly, unlike US and MRI, radionuclide techniques are not operator dependent and provide high reproducibility, including quantitative measurements. Furthermore, unlike echography, radionuclide methods allow a panoramic analysis and are now the easiest way to perform whole body studies. A further major advantage of nuclear medicine is its feasibility in all patients, as it is not constrained by methodological difficulties or a need for previous hematochemical data. In fact, although ionizing radiation is contraindicated in pregnant or pediatric patients, radionuclide procedures can be performed in these subjects, which is clearly cost effective. Whereas it is rarely used in pregnant subjects and justified in only exceptional cases, it must be pointed out that the indications in pediatrics are numerous, where the low radiation dose and the high clinical gain create a primary role in many oncologic and non-oncologic diseases [16].

Although functional imaging is also considered "traditional" radiography, along with CT, US, and MRI when using contrast media or advanced/implemented techniques, nuclear medicine is unique over all the other procedures because it is solely a functional method. In other words, the image in nuclear medicine is only feasible in living beings because of differences in concentration and is never dependent on structural elements [17]. Unlike morphostructural techniques where pathology is the gold standard, nuclear medicine is based on a pathophysiological premise, meaning that the clinical information it provides focuses on a search for altered function. Thus, diagnosis can be made earlier than with methods based on pathological changes that occur later and the information provided is more connected with prognosis and therapy. Conversely, nuclear medicine cannot provide a rigorous anatomical definition and is therefore unable to correctly locate a lesion or reliably define a structural change [18].

To reiterate more specifically the ideas we have already discussed, the best way to describe nuclear medicine is to introduce the concept of "biological tracers" in a scenario in which homeostasis is the object.

We are made up of molecules (and cells) that interact dynamically with the goal of biological equilibrium, called homeostasis. In the large majority of cases, disease may result in an imbalance of homeostasis and can therefore be analyzed and/or detected using biological tracers of the molecular/cellular process. In other words, we can trace a molecular kinetic using a "tracing" molecule that behaves in a similar way to native molecules but is marked with a label detectable by an external probe. The label used depends on the DI technique used: undergoing a change in density for radiography and CT; modifying the magnetic field for MRI; improving the US signal in echography; emitting light in optical imaging; and releasing ionizing radiation in nuclear medicine. To correctly and harmlessly trace a molecular kinetic in humans, it is crucial that a very small ponderal amount of tracer is used, preferably in the range of pico- to nanomoles or less. This is necessary to avoid both toxicity and interference with molecular processes. In the large majority of biological molecular systems, this is possible almost exclusively with optical imaging and nuclear medicine, which are the most sensitive and therefore require the smallest ponderal amount of tracer. Nevertheless, although optical imaging is probably the best imaging procedure in the evaluation of genomics, proteomics, and so on, its inability to detect light signals at depth is a disadvantage. Therefore, although optical imaging may be very useful in animal research or in evaluating superficial lesions, it cannot answer relevant diagnostic questions such as the presence of liver or bone metastases. Therefore, its clinical role in humans could be limited to study of (at least partially) territories such as the skin, eye, gastrointestinal mucosa, or organ surfaces with endoscopic or intra-surgical procedures. Therefore, although nuclear medicine is the only procedure that can widely define a disease at the molecular level, possible improvements in its ability to evaluate molecular processes involve the spatial resolution of machines and the availability of suitable radiotracers. Thus, although the ability to diagnose mutations is currently only used in animal research, old gamma cameras were able to differentiate thyroid carcinoma in humans via identification of the iodine symporter gene as far back as the 1940s, when nuclear medicine began.

Another important concept is that of the radiocompound (or radiopharmaceutical), defined as a complex constituted with a molecular structure chosen based on the specific clinical need to analyze a particular organ or disease [19]. The radiocompound comprises a vector that determines the molecular kinetics of the entire compound, to which is added a radionuclide emitting gamma rays (or positrons, each of which is transformed by annihilation in two gamma rays with the same energy and direction, but opposite verse). These radiocompounds localize based on a specific pathophysiological mechanism and therefore may trace different functions. Thus, we can distinguish a large series of radiotracers with a different uptake mechanism determined by metabolism, receptors, perfusion, immunological pattern, organ characteristics, and so on [20]. Therefore, as an example, when studying liver diseases, we can use radiocolloids to evaluate the reticuloendothelial system, radio-dyes to study the hepatobiliary system, metabolic agents to detect early metastases, radiolabeled red blood cells to diagnose angiomas, somatostatin analogues to evaluate neuroendocrine tumors, and so on.

As it is possible to radiolabel almost all molecules and cells, nuclear medicine can help us study the most important pathophysiological events with procedures that can determine an early diagnosis; correctly analyze viable tissue, which is very important in the diagnosis of recurrence and/or to guide biopsy; define prognostic information and a closer connection with therapeutic strategies; and better define the target for radiotherapy [21]. Furthermore, we can obtain very relevant information for pathology, mainly in follow-up studies, such as defining activity in chronic diseases, the evidence of an escape phenomenon in neoplasia if a biological target

detected at the first diagnosis disappears, and demonstration of reaching a target despite biological obstacles such as the blood–brain barrier [22].

In this context, the best results from a clinical viewpoint are currently obtained with PET using fluorine-18 (F-18) fluorodeoxyglucose (FDG), probably the most relevant diagnostic imaging procedure in oncology today. Moreover, a large series of radionuclide studies are available that also use gamma emitters, which are very important in routine clinical practice, for both oncology and non-oncology requests.

Hybrid Machines

As previously reported, morphostructural and functional imaging methods have substantial complementary advantages and disadvantages. In particular, morphostructural methods can visualize millimetric (and sometimes submillimetric) lesions, easily managing a regional analysis and thereby enabling correct definition of the relationship of a lesion with its spatial context. This is very useful, for example, for regional staging and/or defining a surgical recruitment while also considering relationships with vessels and nerves [23]. Furthermore, because of their high spatial resolution, morphostructural procedures can correctly localize a lesion and obtain differential information based on pathology as the gold standard. A further advantage relates to the possibility of directing a biopsy or intervention via easy detection of anatomical landmarks. Conversely, nuclear medicine is based on a pathophysiological premise, frequently enabling earlier diagnosis and a better connection with prognosis and therapy. Nevertheless, radionuclide procedures cannot correctly localize lesions and/or to make a correct regional analysis.

Some years ago, digital imaging signaled a great improvement in DI. One of the most important achievements has been obtaining fusion imaging between computerized studies (geometrically overlapping), including those obtained with different techniques. Thus, the overlap between functional information provided by PET–FDG and the morphostructural data provided by CT may enable the correct location of lesions previously seen with PET and thereby significantly improve diagnostic accuracy [24].

The arrival of so-called hybrid machines signaled a further major technological improvement. The most widely available tools are systems that combine PET (or SPECT) and CT within the same gantry. The first combination PET–MRI scanners are now available and promise to increase information between function (PET) and structure (MRI), with further functional contributions provided by MR [25]. In other words, the combination of PET–MRI means it is possible to not only better analyze demyelinating cerebral diseases or better detect and define lesions located in the pelvis, head, and neck but also to create new functional images that include metabolic information acquired by PET and an angiogenic pattern or biochemical process evidenced by MRI or MRS. Both these functional images will be perfectly located based on the morphostructural data given by MRI [26].

Lessons Learned

The primary and interactive role of in vivo DI compared with pathology can be easily understood, as it is explained in multitudes of books and papers. An understanding of the relevance of this interrelationship is a mandatory and fundamental educational matter for a modern physician. Less evident is the understanding of the possible role of DI by means of machines routinely used in clinical practice to help the pathologist post mortem. In fact, the knowledge of this interrelationship is mainly limited to specialized conditions, such as those concerning pathologists working on autopsies, not widespread knowledge for the "standard" physician.

Of course, in this field, the role of DI may be limited to morphostructural techniques such as standard CT and MRI, as nuclear medicine and all other functional studies can only contribute information from living beings.

As an example of how morphostructural information provided by such machines can assist the pathologist working in autopsies, the next chapter details our experience with CT and MRI in the definition of anatomical features of cephalothoracopagi.

References

1. Wears RL. Risk, radiation, and rationality. Ann Emerg Med. 2011;58(1):9–11.
2. Mitchell R. An overview: radiography for the imaging technician. Biomed Instrum Technol. 2012;46 (3):202–6.
3. Cronin P, Dwamena BA, Kelly AM, Carlos RC. Solitary pulmonary nodules: meta-analytic comparison of cross-sectional imaging modalities for diagnosis of malignancy. Radiology. 2008;246 (3):772–82.
4. Eisenberg RL. The role of abdominal radiography in the evaluation of the non trauma emergency patient: new thoughts on an old problem. Radiology. 2008;248 (3):715–6.
5. Pasternak JJ, Williamson EE. Clinical pharmacology, uses, and adverse reactions of iodinated contrast agents: a primer for the non-radiologist. Mayo Clin Proc. 2012;87(4):390–402.
6. Thomsen HS. Recent hot topics in contrast media. Eur Radiol. 2011;21(3):492–5.
7. Ilangovan R, Burling D, George A, Gupta A, Marshall M, Taylor SA. CT enterography: review of technique and practical tips. Br J Radiol. 2012;85 (1015):876–86.
8. Osborn EA, Jaffer FA. The year in molecular imaging. JACC Cardiovasc Imaging. 2012;5(3):317–28.
9. Sabarudin A, Sun Z, Ng KH. A systematic review of radiation dose associated with different generations of multidetector CT coronary angiography. J Med Imaging Radiat Oncol. 2012;56(1):5–17.
10. Anzidei M, Napoli A, Zini C, Kirchin MA, Catalano C, Passariello R. Malignant tumours of the small intestine: a review of histopathology, multidetector CT and MRI aspects. Br J Radiol. 2011;84(1004):677–90.
11. Aggeli C, Felekos I, Siasos G, Tousoulis D, Stefanadis C. Ultrasound contrast agents: updated data on safety profile. Curr Pharm Des. 2012;18(15):2253–8.
12. Bhargava P, Dighe MK, Lee JH, Wang C. Multimodality imaging of ureteric disease. Radiol Clin North Am. 2012;50(2):271–99.
13. Taffel M, Haji-Momenian S, Nikolaidis P, Miller FH. Adrenal imaging: a comprehensive review. Radiol Clin North Am. 2012;50(2):219–43.
14. Verma S, Turkbey B, Muradyan N, Rajesh A, Cornud F, Haider MA, Choyke PL, Harisinghani M. Overview of dynamic contrast-enhanced MRI in

prostate cancer diagnosis and management. AJR Am J Roentgenol. 2012;198(6):1277–88.

15. Lambregts DM, Maas M, Cappendijk VC, Prompers LM, Mottaghy FM, Beets GL, Beets-Tan RG. Whole-body diffusion-weighted magnetic resonance imaging: current evidence in oncology and potential role in colorectal cancer staging. Eur J Cancer. 2011;47(14):2107–16.

16. Mansi L. Nuclear medicine is to Fukushima as drug is to poison: el sueño de la razón produce monstruos. Eur J Nucl Med Mol Imaging. 2012;39(2):369–72.

17. Mansi L. The absolute (quantitative): dialogue between St. Thomas and Lord Kelvin: interview with Stephen L. Bacharach, as recorded by Luigi Mansi. Eur J Nucl Med Mol Imaging. 2008;35(9):1725–8.

18. Mansi L. Ich bin ein Molekularmediziner (how much CT and nuclear medicine in molecular CT?). Eur J Nucl Med Mol Imaging. 2009;36(3):531–2.

19. Herrmann K, Benz MR, Krause BJ, Pomykala KL, Buck AK, Czernin J. (18)F-FDG-PET/CT in evaluating response to therapy in solid tumors: where we are and where we can go. Q J Nucl Med Mol Imaging. 2011;55(6):620–32.

20. Gulyás B, Halldin C. New PET radiopharmaceuticals beyond FDG for brain tumor imaging. Q J Nucl Med Mol Imaging. 2012;56(2):173–90.

21. Cuccurullo V, Cascini G, Rossi A, Tamburrini O, Rotondo A, Mansi L. Pathophysiological premises to radiotracers for bone metastases. Q J Nucl Med Mol Imaging. 2011;55(4):353–73.

22. Ambrosini V, Tomassetti P, Franchi R, Fanti S. Imaging of NETs with PET radiopharmaceuticals. Q J Nucl Med Mol Imaging. 2010;54(1):16–23.

23. Götz L, Spehl TS, Weber WA, Grosu AL. PET and SPECT for radiation treatment planning. Q J Nucl Med Mol Imaging. 2012;56(2):163–72.

24. Rice SL, Roney CA, Daumar P, Lewis JS. The next generation of positron emission tomography radiopharmaceuticals in oncology. Semin Nucl Med. 2011;41(4):265–82.

25. Buchbender C, Heusner TA, Lauenstein TC, Bockisch A, Antoch G. Oncologic PET/MRI, part 1: tumors of the brain, head and neck, chest, abdomen, and pelvis. J Nucl Med. 2012;53(6):928–38.

26. Mansi L, Ciarmiello A, Cuccurullo V. PET/MRI and the revolution of the third eye. Eur J Nucl Med Mol Imaging. 2012;39(10):1519–24.

Clinical Imaging Experimental Example in Pathology

11

Graziella Di Grezia, Roberto Grassi, Maria Paola Belfiore, and Luigi Mansi

Introduction

As reported in the previous chapter, diagnostic imaging may significantly and interactively help pathologists in many ways with its ability to detect and characterize human diseases ante- and postmortem using non-invasive or minimally invasive approaches. In particular, a contribution relevant to autopsy is the ability to study skeletal diseases and calcifications, including malformations, injuries, foreign bodies, and gas accumulations [1–3].

Advances in medical imaging and the constant development of three-dimensional (3D) reconstructions have resulted in images that are easily understandable, even without radiology training. They have also further stimulated the creation of a bridge over the compartmentalization of disciplines, perpetuating and reinforcing the legacy of a multidisciplinary approach. The ability to bring together researchers from different specialties (from biology and anatomy to radiology, pathology, and forensic pathology) may improve the core of modern "tailored" medicine, which focuses on the patient rather than the disease.

G. Di Grezia (✉) • R. Grassi • M.P. Belfiore • L. Mansi
Sezione Scientifica di Radiodiagnostica, Radioterapia
e Medicina Nucleare. Dipartimento Medico Chirurgico di
Internistica Clinica e Sperimentale "F. MAGRASSI"
e "A. LANZARA", Seconda Università degli Studi di
Napoli, Naples, Italy
e-mail: graziella.digrezia@libero.it

Moreover, an interdisciplinary approach and the ability to choose between different morpho-functional methods and multi-planar reconstructions allows us to overcome the previous system, which was based on the concept of a "better diagnosis for each examination" obtained using a sum of "two-dimensional (2D) thinking" and was less able to provide the best final answer. We now have access to more information enriched by the interactive contribution of each protagonist on the diagnostic tree.

In particular, close collaboration between the pathologist and the radiologist may be necessary for reliable sampling, accurate diagnostic assessment, and a successful outcome [4]. To demonstrate how the pathologist may find diagnostic imaging information useful, we provide an example from our experience with cephalothoracopagi.

Introduction to Cephalothoracopagus

Conjoined twins have fascinated humankind for a long time. Until recently, however, description of this condition has been limited to the dissection of nonviable cases or to the descriptions of external features and skeletal analysis allowed by traditional standard X-ray imaging [5, 6].

The prenatal diagnosis of cephalothoracopagus is very important so that parents may be counseled, and a prognosis may be defined, as

F.M. Sacerdoti et al. (eds.), *Advanced Imaging Techniques in Clinical Pathology*,
Current Clinical Pathology, DOI 10.1007/978-1-4939-3469-0_11

these could support the interruption of pregnancy. The first diagnostic approach is usually 2D ultrasound (US). This is the most important imaging method for the diagnosis of fetal malformations as it is cheap, poses no risk to the pregnancy or the pregnant woman, is widely available, and can be conducted at the bedside. The limitations of US include reverberation artifacts and the inability to visualize fetal intracranial anomalies, meaning the sensitivity for detecting cerebral cortical malformations or small destructive lesions of the cerebrum is low [7–9]. Power Doppler ultrasonography in combination with high-definition color Doppler may further help in the visualization of vascular structures and complex vascular malformations. Similarly, echocardiography should be used to establish the degree of cardiac conjunction and associated structural heart abnormalities.

Computed tomography (CT) provides excellent anatomic detail, at first of bones and calcified tissues and then also organ position, shared viscera, and vascular anatomy.

Magnetic resonance imaging (MRI) is the best modality to provide detailed imaging of fetuses with complex anomalies, especially in late pregnancy. In particular, ultrafast imaging sequences have revolutionized fetal imaging, providing the most effective contribution to neuroradiological examination.

Contrast-enhanced imaging using different procedures also enables the evaluation of gastrointestinal and urogenital tracts and may improve assessment of a shared liver based on anatomy and vascularization.

Although cephalothoracopagi can be classified based on the site of union (ventral, dorsal, or more rare forms of union), each set of conjoined twins is unique. Therefore, an individually specific imaging strategy is mandatory to accurately define anatomic fusion, vascular anomalies, and other associated abnormalities, as an important base for correct surgical planning and reliable prognostic information.

In addition, 3D reconstruction of US, CT, and MRI images permit direct spatial visualization of fetal malformations, which is especially helpful for non-radiologists, although 3D images have not been proven to be better than 2D and axial images in this diagnostic situation.

We present our experience in studying very rare conjoined cephalothoracopagi (joined at the head and/or at the thorax) using CT and MRI. It was possible to study skeletal and visceral structures to obtain precious details for accurate understanding of diagnostic images, and for a better etiological understanding of malformations [10].

Six cephalothoracopagi twins were acquired by the Museum of Anatomy of the Second University of Naples in the period 1950–1980 and preserved in formalin. We conducted CT and MRI scanning of these twins at our diagnostic imaging department. We performed CT scans using a four-slice multi-detector CT scanner from head to feet and used a commercially available workstation for 3D volume rendering. MRI studies were acquired with a 1.5 T machine, using head, knee, or wrist receiver, according to the fetal size, and TSE T2-W axial/TSE T1-W axial sequences.

Macroscopic details of the fetuses, as shown by CT and MRI, demonstrated that the samples were well preserved. The internal organs were well represented. Brain regions showed some artifacts (regions of vacuolization), probably because they had been preserved for a long time.

In the following paragraphs, we describe all six cases individually (Table 11.1):

- Cephalothoracopagus deradelphous
  The two fetuses are joined at head; the face is shared by the two, one half belonging to one fetus and one half to the other. The two vertebral columns and spinal cords are completely independent and diverge inferiorly. The arms and the legs of the two fetuses are well formed and independent.
- Cephalothoracopagus deradelphous (Fig. 11.1)
  The two fetuses are joined at the head; the visceral structures are evident. The subarachnoid spaces appear dilated, possibly due to the long-term fixation of the specimen. At the neurocranial level, the brain shows a composite structure with a very complex ventricular system: a single large central cavity is evident.

Table 11.1 Macroscopic details of the six conjoined twins as shown by computed tomography (CT) and magnetic resonance imaging (MRI)

		Eyes	Nose	Ears	Oral cavity	Vertebral column	Spinal cord	Arms	Legs	Tracheal system	Superior GI tract	Inferior GI tract
1	Cephalothoracopagus deradelphous	2	1	2	1	2	2	4	4	2	1	2
2	Cephalothoracopagus deradelphous	2	1	2	1	2	2	4	4	2	1	2
3	Cephalothoracopagus iniop	2	1	4	1	2	2	4	4	2	1	2
4	Cephalothoracopagus iniop	3	1	4	1	2	2	4	4	2	1	2
5	Cephalothoracopagus deradelphous diprosopous	3	2	2	2	2	2	4	4	2	1	2
6	Cephalothoracopagus symmetricus (Janiceps)	4	2	4	2	2	2	4	4	1	1	2

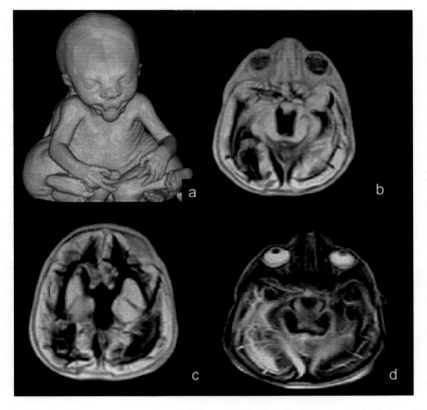

Fig. 11.1 Cephalothoracopagus deradelphous. (**a**) CT shows the two fetuses joined at the head. (**b** and **c**) MRI shows a composite neurocranial structure with a complex ventricular system. (**d**) The nasal cavities show an initial attempt at duplication

Closer inspection reveals four parallel lateral ventricles. The lower part of the brain is formed by two separate brainstems and spinal cords. The ocular cavities are well shaped, and two separate optic nerves can be observed. The nasal cavities show an initial attempt at duplication; therefore, the nasal septum is duplicated with a shared middle nasal cavity. The oral cavities are also very complex and highly deformed in their shape because of the presence of a septum. There is only one large pharyngeal cavity that continues in a single esophagus, shared by the two fetuses, but two tracheal systems lie on a plane perpendicular to the plane that passes through the vertebral columns. The lower airways are not represented in the MRI study. Similar to the skull, the heart is a composite structure, located to one side of the two fetuses, with four cavities. Four undeveloped lungs can be observed on one side of the chest. While two livers are evident, the esophagus continues to a single stomach and upper gastrointestinal system. The lower intestinal tract is doubled, similar to the posterior structures of the abdominal cavity (kidneys and rectum).

• Cephalothoracopagus iniop (Fig. 11.2)
The two fetuses are joined at the head and chest. The fusion of the two cranial parts of each twin is incomplete. In fact, the single head shows a composite face on one side, and two ears on the other. This might be due to the enlargement of the cranial vault. This phenomenon is called "concentration of the facial structures" and entails hypotrophy of one face when compared with a perfect Janus. The face is well shaped but is shared by the twins; it is a composite structure with one-half belonging to one fetus and one-half to the other. Independent vertebral columns and spinal cords diverge inferiorly, whereas the arms and legs are well formed and independent.

• Cephalothoracopagus iniop
The two fetuses are joined at the head and chest. The single head shows a composite face on one side and two ears on the other side. Although the brain is not well preserved, it is possible to observe several structures. The subarachnoid spaces appear dilated, possibly due to the long-term fixation of the specimen. A single great falx separates the upper cranial cavity into two halves, forming an angle in the center. From this point, a second separation divides the opposing frontal poles on the side with the well-shaped face. The face is sufficiently well defined: two eyes and a well-shaped nasal cavity can be clearly recognized. The optic nerves converge toward the composite midline, but do not form a chiasm [11]. On the side with two external ears, MRI also reveals a single empty ocular cavity (cyclopia) and a chiasm. At the neurocranial level, the brain is a composite structure with a

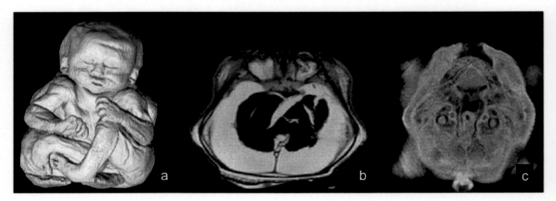

Fig. 11.2 Cephalothoracopagus iniop. (**a**) CT shows the two fetuses joined at the head and chest. The fusion of the two cranial parts of the two fetuses is incomplete. In fact, MRI (**b** and **c**) shows the single head with a composite face on one side and two ears on the other

very complex ventricular system: it seems to display a single large central cavity, but closer inspection reveals four parallel lateral ventricles. The lower part of the brain is formed by two separate brainstems and spinal cords. The ocular cavities are well shaped, and two separate optic nerves can be observed. The nasal cavities present an initial attempt at duplication: therefore, the nasal septum is duplicated with a shared middle nasal cavity. The oral cavities are also very complex and highly deformed in their shape due to the presence of a septum. There is only large pharyngeal cavity that continues in a single esophagus shared by the fetuses, but two tracheal systems lie on a plane perpendicular to the plane that passes through the vertebral columns. The pericardium, pleural, and peritoneal folds are well represented, whereas

heart and lungs are not preserved. However, there is only one pericardial cavity, suggesting the presence of only one heart. There are two livers, highly dystrophic, with their triangular ligaments well preserved. The kidneys are hypotrophic. The terminal part of the intestinal tract can be easily traced.

- Cephalothoracopagus deradelphous diprosopous (Fig. 11.3)
  The two fetuses are joined at the head, sharing half a face and the chest. Two vertebral columns and spinal cords are completely independent and diverge inferiorly. The arms and the legs of the two fetuses are well formed and independent.
- Cephalothoracopagus symmetricus (Janiceps) (Fig. 11.4)
  The two fetuses are joined at the head and chest. The fusion of the two cranial parts of

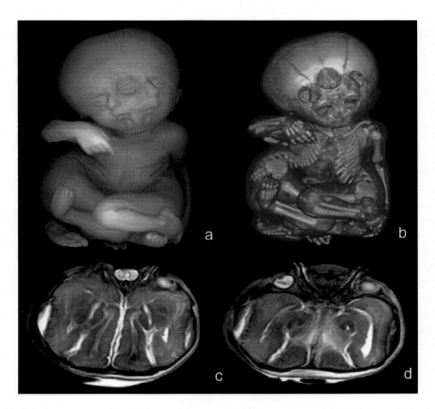

Fig. 11.3 Cephalothoracopagus deradelphous diprosopus. (**a** and **b**) CT shows the two fetuses joined at the head, sharing half a face, and the chest. (**c** and **d**) MRI shows incomplete division of structures of the splanchnocranium, resulting in three eyes (one eye is shared)

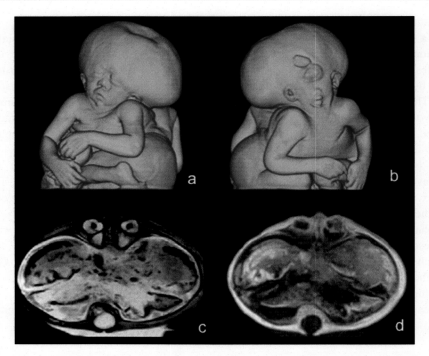

Fig. 11.4 Cephalothoracopagus symmetricus (Janiceps). The two fetuses are joined at the head and chest, as shown by CT (**a** and **b**); MRI shows two composite faces on the two sides (**c** and **d**); one side is cyclopic

the twins is symmetrical. In fact, the single head shows two composite faces on two sides. This might be due to the enlargement of the cranial vault. On one side, the face is cyclopean. This phenomenon is called "concentration of the facial structures" and consists of the hypotrophy of one face when compared with a perfect Janus. The face is well-shaped but shared by the twins and therefore is a composite structure with one-half to one fetus and one-half to the other. The sphenoid represents the center of the mass of the single head, appearing as a very deformed structure shared by the fetuses. A single pituitary fossa communicates with the pharyngeal cavity. A single, greatly enlarged, rhinopharyngeal cavity continues in a unique enlarged oral cavity with two opposite tongues. The arms and legs of the two fetuses are well formed and independent.

Discussion

Conjoined twins are believed to be monozygotic monochorionic twins of the same sex and identical chromosomal patterns [5–7], with an embryogenesis first hypothesized as dependent on the fusion of two different embryos [8, 9]. Successive hypotheses were instead based on the incomplete fission in the early stages of embryo development [10, 11], although, very recently, the fusion hypothesis has been re-proposed [12]. Unfortunately, this theory does not account for parasitic twins and, unless there is an associated event, does not explain the abnormalities in the formation of the fused and non-fused organs [13]. At present, there is no evidence for linkage between chromosomal abnormalities, mutant gene disorders, or specific genetic loci and predisposition to conjoined twinning; their formation appears rather to be the effect of random processes, probably regulated by environmental factors [8] and possibly dependent on the age of the mother. Single reports of changes in the chromosomes in cases of conjoined twins could therefore be considered spurious associations [14].

Starting from our experience, first based on morphostructural analysis of Janiceps (Cephalothoracopagus symmetricus) [15–17], we subsequently decided to use diagnostic imaging to gain a better understanding of its integrative role with respect to pathology in this very specific field. In our paper published in 2004 in *Radiographics* [18], we provide a deeper and wider analysis of the most important issues concerning cephalothoracopagi.

We conclude this chapter stating that our experience clearly supports diagnostic imaging as a primary aid for the pathologist. Whereas the role of diagnostic imaging in living beings is supportive, CT and MRI play the major role in study of the corpse. It is also evident by our reported experience that CT has primacy in evaluating organs with low hydrogen content, such as bone and lungs and/or structures that are calcified or that contain gases. Conversely, MRI is superior when improved contrast is required for evaluating territories with low (proton) density differences between adjacent tissues, such as in the brain and pelvis, spinal cord, tendons, and ligaments, because of the density and composition of the tissues.

Both CT and MRI scanners can generate multiple 2D cross sections (slices) of tissue and 3D reconstructions. Unlike CT, which uses only X-ray attenuation to generate image contrast, MRI has a long list of properties that may be used to generate image contrast. By varying scanning parameters, tissue contrast can be altered and enhanced in various ways to detect different features.

MRI can generate cross-sectional images in any plane (including oblique planes). CT was previously limited to acquiring images in the axial (or near axial) plane and were previously called computed axial tomography (CAT) scans. However, the development of multi-detector CT scanners with near-isotropic resolution enables the CT scanner to produce data that can be retrospectively reconstructed in any plane with minimal loss of image quality.

While CT provides good spatial resolution (the ability to distinguish as separate two structures at an arbitrarily small distance from each other), MRI provides comparable resolution with far better contrast resolution (the ability to distinguish differences between two arbitrarily similar but not identical tissues). The basis of this ability is the complex library of pulse sequences that the modern medical MRI scanner includes, each of which is optimized to provide image contrast based on the chemical sensitivity of MRI.

For example, with particular echo time (TE) and repetition time (TR) values, basic parameters of image acquisition, a sequence may take on the property of T2 weighting. On a T2-weighted scan, tissues containing fat, water, or fluid are bright (most modern T2 sequences are actually fast T2 sequences). Damaged tissue tends to develop edema, which makes a T2-weighted sequence sensitive for pathology, and pathologic tissue is generally distinguishable from normal tissue. With the addition of an additional radiofrequency pulse and additional manipulation of the magnetic gradients, a T2-weighted sequence can be converted to a fluid-attenuated inversion recovery (FLAIR) sequence, in which free water becomes dark but edematous tissues remain bright. This sequence in particular is currently the most sensitive way to evaluate the brain for demyelinating diseases, such as multiple sclerosis.

CT is the preferred modality for cancer and pneumonia and after abnormal chest X-rays. Bleeding in the brain, especially from injury, is better seen via CT than MRI. CT displays the inner auditory canals well and shows organ tear and organ injury quickly and efficiently. Broken bones and the vertebral bodies of the spine are better visualized on CT, but injury to the spinal cord itself is displayed far better on MRI than on CT.

CT is far superior for visualizing the lungs and organs in the chest cavity between the lungs. MRI is not a good tool for visualizing the chest or lungs at all. Any decision over whether to use

MRI or CT scanning depends on what needs to be visualized and the reason for the test.

Although both CT and MRI each provide relevant information, the best results are obtained when they are used in conjunction.

References

1. Sochor MR, Trowbridge MJ, Boscak A, Maino JC, Maio RF. Postmortem computed tomography as an adjunct to autopsy for analyzing fatal motor vehicle crash injuries: results of a pilot study. J Trauma. 2008;65(3):659–65.
2. Aghayev E, Sonnenschein M, Jackowski C, et al. Postmortem radiology of fatal hemorrhage: measurements of cross-sectional areas of major blood vessels and volumes of aorta and spleen on MDCT and volumes of heart chambers on MRI. AJR Am J Roentgenol. 2006;187:209–15.
3. Jackowski C, Thali M, Sonnenschein M, et al. Visualization and quantification of air embolism structure by processing postmortem MSCT data. J Forensic Sci. 2004;49:1339–42.
4. Bolliger SA, Filograna L, Spendlove D, et al. Postmortem imaging-guided biopsy as an adjuvant to minimally invasive autopsy with CT and postmortem angiography: a feasibility study. AJR Am J Roentgenol. 2010;195(5):1051–105.
5. O'Neill JA. Conjoined twins. In: O'Neill JA, Rowe MI, Grosfiled JL, editors. Pediatric surgery. St. Louis, MO: Mosby; 1998. p. 1925–38.
6. Hoyle RM. Surgical separation of conjoined twins. Surg Gynecol Obstet. 1990;170:549–62.
7. Zimmermann AA. Embryologic and anatomic considerations of conjoined twins. Birth Defects. 1967;3:18–27.
8. Steinman G. Mechanisms of twinning. V. Conjoined twins, stem cells and the calcium model. J Reprod Med. 2002;47:313–21.
9. Eichhorn K. Zurgenese des cephalothoracopagus monosymmetros. Acta Anat. 1969;73:255–71.
10. Duhamle B, Haegel P, Pagès R. Morphogenèse pathologique. Paris: Masson & C.ie editeurs; 1966.
11. Herring SW, Rowlatt UF. Anatomy and embryology in cephalothoracopagus twins. Teratology. 1981;23:159–73.
12. Sperber GH, Machin GA. Microscopic study of the midline determinants in Janiceps twins. Birth Defects Orig Artic Ser. 1987;23:243–75.
13. Spencer R. Theoretical and analytical embryology of conjoined twins, part 1: embryogenesis. Clin Anat. 2000;13:36–53.
14. Delprado WI, Baird PJ. Cephalothoracopagus syncephalus: a case report with previously unreported anatomical abnormalities and chromosomal analysis. Teratology. 1984;29:1–9.
15. Viggiano D, Pirolo L, Cappabianca S, Passiatore C. Testing the model of optic chiasm formation in human beings. Brain Res Bull. 2002;59:111–5.
16. Pirolo L, Viggiano D, Amoroso A, Passiatore C. Inferior vena cava duplications with reference to venous asymmetries. Ital J Anat Embryol. 2002;107:169–75.
17. Viggiano D, Cappabianca S, Passiatore C. Is our brain changing? Antropologica et Prehistorica. 2003;114:1–6.
18. Grassi R, Esposito V, Scaglione M, Cirillo M, Cappabianca S, Guglielmi G, Sasso FS, Rotondo A. Multi-detector row CT for depicting anatomic features of cephalothoracopagus varieties: revised approach. Radiographics. 2004;24(5):e21.

Ultrasound in the Evaluation of Cutaneous Diseases

12

Maria Paola Belfiore, Roberto Grassi, Graziella Di Grezia, Vincenzo Cuccurullo, Claudia Rossi, and Luigi Mansi

Introduction

Ultrasound (US) represents a primary tool in diagnostic imaging (DI) in humans, with technical capabilities influenced by physical issues, such as US frequency, expressed in megahertz. Higher-frequency ultrasound (HFUS) (20–100 MHz) provides better resolution, albeit to the detriment of tissue penetration. Therefore, HFUS may be proposed for evaluating the skin, as it can visualize the dermis (20 MHz) and even the epidermis (50–100 MHz), with a spatial resolution on the order of microns. For these reasons, and based on our own experience, we report major technical issues and clinical examples demonstrating the possible clinical role of HFUS in studying cutaneous diseases.

We first define the scope; then we introduce the diagnostic scenario, defining spaces in which HFUS could fulfill a clinical role. Therefore, after a short premise defining the (limited) role of DI in the study of skin lesions, we briefly present the most important standard procedures and devices.

The primary aim of the chapter focuses on HFUS, distinguished as a technique that is able to assist in studies of the skin, with the possibility of a high cost-effectiveness ratio. After describing the technique, we provide some examples of normal skin and then some of the most common and/or clinically interesting cutaneous diseases, supported by significant images. The value of our contribution in this area is in the comparison, when possible, of HFUS results with pathological data. The chapter concludes with the lessons learned and an up-to-date bibliography.

Scope

Technological evolution guided by research in animals has been and is a relevant motivation for the technical implementation of DI scanners in humans. Improvements gained in preclinical magnetic resonance imaging (MRI) or hybrid machines have been transferred to use in humans, through the solution of further complex and expensive problems relating to the need to produce equipment in larger dimensions. Conversely, issues regarding the acquisition of new and improved probes for US first proposed in preclinical research have been followed by the production of probes that may be used in humans without any further modification.

In this chapter, which focuses on the diagnosis of skin diseases, we center our analysis

M.P. Belfiore (✉) • R. Grassi • G. Di Grezia • V. Cuccurullo • C. Rossi • L. Mansi
Sezione Scientifica di Radiodiagnostica, Radioterapia e Medicina Nucleare, Dipartimento Medico Chirurgico di Internistica Clinica e Sperimentale "F. MAGRASSI" e "A. LANZARA", Seconda Università degli Studi di Napoli, Naples, Italy
e-mail: mariapaolabelfiore@gmail.com

© Springer Science+Business Media New York 2016
F.M. Sacerdoti et al. (eds.), *Advanced Imaging Techniques in Clinical Pathology*, Current Clinical Pathology, DOI 10.1007/978-1-4939-3469-0_12

on information obtainable with HFUS. To better define its interest for pathologists, images acquired using this new device are compared with corresponding histopathological data. The core argument is briefly preceded by a discussion of the whole diagnostic scenario, including the most important techniques used in skin diseases, classified in terms of invasiveness, cost, and technical complexity.

General Premise

The Diagnostic Scenario in Which HFUS Could Find a Clinical Role in the Evaluation of Skin Lesions

In the diagnostic scenario, the role of a procedure is dependent not only on its capability, but also on the abilities of alternative techniques. Furthermore, clinical significance may be found via a favorable cost effectiveness compared with methods answering the same question or replying to different queries, as well as in those better defining a differential diagnosis or producing a closer connection with prognosis and therapy. Superficial skin lesions generally characterized by a low thickness are an unfavorable field of analysis for standard DI procedures. This is because of the intrinsic limitations of DI and the availability of alternative techniques with better cost effectiveness. Nevertheless, computed tomography (CT), MRI, positron emission tomography (PET) with F-18 fluorodeoxyglucose (FDG), and the sentinel node technique as a precursor to radio-guided surgery in melanoma may find a clinical role, though one mainly limited to the staging and re-staging of oncologic lesions. Conversely, the role of DI in the first evaluation of a cutaneous lesion is less relevant as it can be more easily and effectively analyzed via alternative diagnostic procedures.

Most Important Standard Procedures and Devices

- *Magnifying lens*: Magnification of surface lesions can be achieved with a handheld lens.

- *Diascopy*: Diascopy is performed by firmly pressing a transparent, hard, flat object (most frequently two microscope slides) on the surface of the skin. This procedure may be helpful in distinguishing erythema from vasodilatation.

- *Wood's Light*: Wood's light ("black light"), first described in 1903, is a useful device for the clinical evaluation of many skin diseases such as pigment disorders, including lentigo maligna, skin infections, and porphyria. Wood's light is strongly absorbed by melanin, meaning it is a useful tool in the evaluation of pigmented lesions. A lesion with an increased concentration of epidermal melanin appears darker than surrounding normal skin, with more contrast than normally discernible via visible light examination.

- *Dermoscopy*: Dermoscopy is a noninvasive technique that uses a handheld instrument (dermoscope) equipped with a light source and magnifying optics. The application of a liquid interface (oil, water, alcohol) to the surface of the skin decreases light reflection by the epidermis. Importantly, dermoscopy increases the clinical diagnostic accuracy of melanoma by 10–20 % and facilitates the differential diagnosis between melanocytic lesions from other pigmented lesions, such as seborrheic keratoses, hemangiomas, and pigmented basal-cell carcinomas (BCCs). This technique has also been applied to the evaluation of inflammatory lesions. Clinicians using dermoscopy began to also appreciate the ability to obtain subsurface diagnostic cues to further improve its diagnostic power.

- *Photography*: One of the most important signs of skin cancer is its history of change. Physicians may frequently encounter situations in which the clinical diagnosis is uncertain, and thus, the presence of baseline "technical and standardized" photographs for comparison can facilitate the decision of whether or not to perform a biopsy.

- *Scrape, pull, and swab*: The scrape, pull, and swab procedure allows sampling of skin lesions as an alternative to biopsy.
- *Biopsy*: Skin biopsy is a fundamental technique in dermatology, as the skin is readily accessible for biopsy. It can be useful to confirm the clinical evaluation when a definitive diagnosis is needed, adding a fundamental clue when the clinical evidence is inconclusive, and also sometimes providing an unsuspected diagnosis [1].

Evolving Technologies (Subsurface Imaging Modalities)

The most important subsurface imaging modalities include optical coherence tomography (OCT), reflectance confocal microscopy (RCM), and skin US.

Rules of thumb that apply to subsurface imaging are that the deeper one sees into the tissue, the lower the image resolution; and longer wavelengths penetrate deeper [2].

- *OCT* produces a 2D vertical image of the skin that is analogous to the above-mentioned B-mode US imaging, except that it utilizes light rather than sound waves. Using the light, the melanin produces an increased light backscatter, making this modality potentially useful for the evaluation of pigmented lesion. Although the standard approach to this technique does not discriminate between benign and malignant lesions, images obtained deeper into the tissue (≥ 1 mm) may allow the assessment of the overall lesion architecture, as well as defining the depth of a tumor's invasion.
- *RCM* allows noninvasive imaging of the epidermis and superficial dermis. Like dermoscopy, RCM acquires images in the horizontal plane, allowing assessment of tissue pathology underlying dermoscopic structures of interest at a cellular-level resolution. Thus, clinicians using dermoscopy may find RCM to be particularly useful.
- *HFUS* is described in the following section.

High-Frequency Ultrasound (HFUS)

Since its initial appearance about 50 years ago, US has become an essential tool for medical diagnosis, as it is a versatile, painless, and noninvasive procedure that can be carried out virtually anywhere and can be readily repeated as it does not involve ionizing radiation. US is based on the fact that tissue components differently impede and reflect acoustic waves. The basic techniques include A-mode, B-mode, and Doppler methods [3]. The standard product is a 2D image (B-scan) of the skin, obtained by displaying the magnitude of acoustic reflection as degrees of brightness. Intermediate ultrasound (medium-frequency US [MFUS]) frequencies (7.5–10 MHz) are routinely used to study subcutaneous structures deeper than 1.5 cm; indications include lymph node evaluation, mainly in melanoma; guidance for needle biopsy; and detection and measurement of choroidal melanoma. Subcutaneous masses are evaluated for size, extent, and consistency, mainly differentiating between solid and cystic lesions.

Recent years have seen the development of HFUS (20–100 MHz) that can visualize the dermis (20 MHz) and even the epidermis (50–100 MHz), although they are not yet widely used in clinical practice. Higher frequencies provide higher resolution, albeit tissue penetration is sacrificed [4]; they are currently under study as a tool to preoperatively assess tumor thickness in melanoma and non-melanoma skin cancer. The hypo-echogenicity of tumors compared with the surrounding dermis forms the basis for image contrast.

Consequently, MFUS and HFUS may find a well-established role in the dermatologic diagnostic work-up of benign and malignant diseases of the skin, given that noninvasive and reliable examination of both superficial and deep cutaneous structures is already possible [5]. A tissue penetration depth of approximately 6–7 mm is possible at a frequency of 20 MHz. In normal skin, the dermis is markedly echogenic and sharply demarcated. Consistency between histology and HFUS results has been well documented, including by statistical analysis.

Therefore, although HFUS will not replace histology in the evaluation of skin cancer, it has already demonstrated its usefulness as a complementary adjunct in surgical planning.

In fact, HFUS enables 3D analyses of tumors in living beings, enabling in-depth examination of the whole skin cancer, and therefore using both visual information acquired via the naked eye and histological analysis, offering a 2D vision and only limited to the biopsied tissue sample.

Current HFUS techniques, based on high variable-frequency US, is an imaging method that produces robust qualitative and quantitative information on skin lesions and surrounding tissues. Moreover, with the inclusion of color Doppler examination, it also provides data on blood flow in real time, enabling, for example, the differentiation between arterial and venous flow, as well as gathering flow velocity and resistance index values for spectral curve analysis. High variable-frequency US equipment is becoming a common tool in DI departments; they cost a similar amount to US tools routinely used in musculoskeletal examinations [6, 7].

HFUS is becoming indispensable in the study of surface structures. In fact, increasing frequencies decrease the power of penetration of the US beam into tissues and increase the resolution power, translating into very defined and detailed images of the skin and subcutaneous tissues, with faithful reproduction of the different layers. To study the superficial tissues with US, a gel must be placed between the probe and the skin, which serves to both slide the probe on the body surface and prevent the interposition of air, which bars the ultrasound beam. For the same reason, the technique can be difficult to perform in anatomical areas such as periocular, perinasal, and perilabial regions, or in the folds of elbows, buttocks, and groin, because of the lack of contact between the probe and the lesion in question. In these cases, a spacer of synthetic material is needed with the dual purpose of flattening the region to be examined and adjusting the lesion to be within the focal area of the probe—a position to allow a more precise and defined image without noise and artifacts [8].

Currently, imaging of the skin is more frequently performed with fixed (non-variable) HFUS. In fixed HFUS, the probe is activated at a single high operating frequency (20–100 MHz) that determines both a high spatial resolution (the capacity to separate two objects in close proximity along the path of the US beam) and a reduced depth of penetration (6–7 mm at 20 MHz, and only 3 mm at 75 MHz). The standard images produced by fixed HFUS are static and do not show deep subcutaneous tissue, vascular pattern, or real-time data on blood flow.

To better understand the method, it is important to remember that US responds to precise rules of physics that cannot be transcended. We know that the diagnostic resolution power of a US probe is directly proportional to its frequency, providing the highest frequencies at the highest resolution and therefore a better definition. Conversely, high frequencies are affected by a smaller penetration capability, thereby defining a smaller field of view. As skin lesions are superficial and frequently small, it logically follows that HFUS probes (usually around 20–25 MHz) are preferred in the study of skin diseases. Conversely, an analysis performed solely with HFUS may be insufficient to fully evaluate, for example, subjects with melanoma, where the presence of metastases in transit, lymph node involvement, and systemic metastases also require lower-frequency probes [9].

US devices with linear probes at 22 MHz are now available and reliably evaluate lesions that are 1 mm. So-called US microscopes that use frequencies from 25 to 50 MHz and can provide very high-detail images, similar to those from a histological preparation or with an OCT are commercially available although less widespread.

Nevertheless, despite the advantages of high-frequency linear probes, the sonographer must choose and correctly set the right device for the specific problem, prioritizing high or medium frequency depending on the clinical and pathologic characteristics of the individual lesion under study. The possibility of integrating a further probe in the analysis, based on the experimental US data, must also be considered. Similarly, when the power color Doppler is used, it must be appropriately preset, choosing a power rate frequency (PRF) and filters to improve detection of the signal.

As previously reported, artifacts are a possible limit to the use of this method in dermatology. To obviate this problem, the sonographers should use an abundant film of gel between the skin and the probe during the US examination to prevent pinching the skin lesion, as the slightest compression causes a loss of signal.

Examples: HFUS Images Compared with Clinical and Histological Features

Normal Skin

To better understand the possible contribution of HFUS to the study of cutaneous lesions, this section briefly introduces the structure and function of the skin. We then provide figures that provide a direct comparison between pathological and US data to help the reader recognize the supporting role that HFUS may occupy in this field.

Structure and Function of the Skin

The skin is a complex organ that simultaneously protects its host from and allows interaction with the environment. As a dynamic integrated arrangement of cells and matrix elements, the skin has different functions: (1) selectively permeable physical barrier, (2) protection against infectious agents, (3) thermoregulation, (4) sensorial activity, (5) protection from ultraviolet (UV), (6) wound repair and regeneration, and (7) outward physical appearance.

Skin function is mediated by one or more of its three major layers—epidermis, dermis, and hypodermis—acting as functional interdependent units (Fig. 12.1a). The outermost epidermis is separated from the dermis by a basal membrane, the dermal–epidermal junction. Below the dermis lies the subcutaneous fat (hypodermis). Epidermal appendages, such as hair follicles and eccrine and apocrine sweat glands, begin in the epidermis but course through to penetrate the dermis and/or epidermis. Blood, lymphatic vessels, and nerves pass through the subcutaneous fat and enter the dermis.

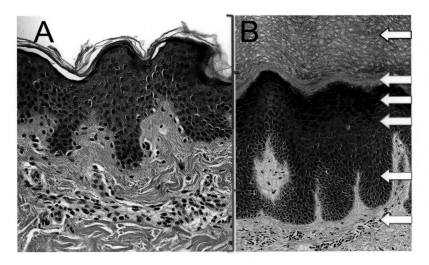

Fig. 12.1 (a) Histological section (hematoxylin eosin) of the skin (in an adult) showing the epidermis (*blue bracket*) and dermis (*red bracket*). (b) Histological section at a greater magnification, individuating the different layers of the epidermis: stratum corneum (*white arrow*) and lucidum (*yellow arrow*), granulosum (*red arrow*), spinosum (*light blue arrow*), and germinative layers (*blue arrow*) are clearly evidenced. The dermis is individuated by the *green arrow*. With permission of the department "Anatomia Patologica," A.O.R.N. San Sebastiano, Caserta, Italy, by courtesy of Carmela Buonomo, MD

The epidermis, including its outer stratum corneum, represents the major component of the physical barrier, with a thickness ranging from 0.4 to 1.5 mm compared with the 1.5 to 4.0 mm full depth of the skin. It comprises both cells and noncellular components. The predominant cells in the epidermis are keratinocytes, which are organized into four layers (basal, spinous, granular, and status corneum), named either for their position or the structural property of the cells (Fig. 12.1a, b). These cells progressively differentiate from proliferative staminal basal cells attached to the epidermal basal membrane to the terminally differentiated keratinized stratum corneum, the outermost layer and barrier. The epidermis also includes specialized non-epidermal cell types such as melanocytes and Langerhans and Merkel cells. The dermal–epidermal junction is a basal membrane zone that forms the interface between the epidermis and dermis.

The dermis is an integrated system of fibrous, filamentous, and cellular connective tissue elements that accommodates nerve, vascular, and lymphatic networks and epidermal-derived appendages and contains many resident cell types, including fibroblasts, macrophages, mast cells, and transient circulating cells of the immune system. The nerve network contains somatic, sensory, and sympathetic autonomic fibers.

The hypodermis is composed of adipocytes (Fig. 12.1a, b), which are the bulk of the cells at this level, and it is organized in lobules defined by septa of fibrous connective tissue. Nerves, blood, and lymphatic vessels are located within the septa and supply the region.

HFUS of the Normal Skin

HFUS probes enable distinction between the three layers of the skin and can also provide wider and better-defined information. In the following section, technical aspects and the clinical potential of HFUS are focused in the study of the skin.

As can be seen by the comparison with pathological images, it is not possible to distinguish the five different layers of the epidermis, but it is possible to discern the transition between epidermis and dermis, and between dermis and hypodermis (Fig. 12.2).

Using 20-MHz US imaging, an uninterrupted hyper-reflecting band can be seen at the boundary between the contact medium and the epidermis. Using 40-MHz transducers, the skin appears composed of several layers (Fig. 12.2a, b). The upper echo-rich line segment corresponds to the water–stratum corneum interface; the echo-rich line segment beneath originates from the stratum corneum–Malpighi's stratum interface. The endostructure of the dermis shows considerable variation in relation to skin site, sex, and age. Its acoustic characteristics depend on the quantity of collagen and orientation of collagen fibers and also on the water content and composition of the base substance [10].

In the following section, we describe some of the most frequent and/or important patterns as seen by HFUS, with a brief preliminary reference to histology and clinics.

HFUS Images Compared with Clinical and Histological Features: Pathological Patterns

Although the goal of this chapter is not the analytical presentation of all cutaneous pathologies, we do present some examples to aid in understanding the abilities and consequently the possible clinical role of HFUS in cutaneous diseases.

Benign Skin Lesions

- *Epidermoid cysts*: At histology, epidermoid cysts are characterized by a thin epithelium and a cavity filled with amorphous debris. The HFUS shows sharp margins and a corpuscular fluid-filled hypo-anechoic lesion with reinforced posterior wall. On color Doppler, the lesion appears avascular.
- *Dermoid cysts*: Deriving from ectodermal elements, they manifest at birth as more or less hard lumps under the skin. The characteristic sonographic feature is the composition of echogenic components with sharp borders and

Fig. 12.2 (**a**) The ultrasonographic image obtained with a 20-MHz probe shows the epidermis (*red arrow*) as a hyper-echogenic and the dermis (*green arrow*) as a hypo-hyperechogenic layer. The *yellow arrow* individuates the hypodermis. (**b**) In the high-resolution ultrasound image (40-MHz probe), the transition between epidermis (*red arrow*) and dermis (*green arrow*), and between dermis and hypodermis (*yellow arrow*), is better evidenced compared with the 20-MHz image

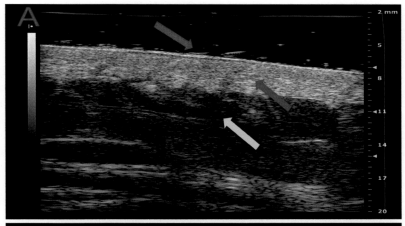
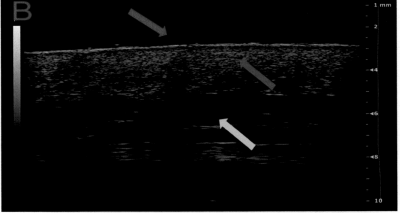

acoustic shadowing. The cyst structure may appear both simple and complex, sometimes including hairs. No second-level investigations are needed unless involvement of nerve structures is suspected.

- *Trichilemmal cysts*: These cysts are a benign variant of proliferative tumors that develop mainly in the skin and in subcutaneous tissue of the scalp, are more frequent in women, and reach various sizes. With HFUS, they appear as a well-circumscribed hypo-echoic mass with calcifications. This is an example of a formation above the muscle planes and more precisely of the galia capitis.

- *Sudoriparous cysts*: The most common sudoriparous cyst is the eccrine or apocrine adenocystoma. It is a bluish lesion affecting adults in the periorbital and neck regions, mainly in the eyelid region, and measuring

generally <1 cm. Sudoriferous cysts also include mucous, ganglion, and deep cysts. The mucous cyst, prevalent in adult women, appears as a solitary nodule, typically located in the vicinity of the distal phalanges of the hands, particularly involving the distal inter-phalangeal joints or the proximal nail fold. The nodule appears as a translucent lump containing a clear, viscous fluid that communicates with the joint cavity; it can deform the fingernail and can also be painful. US shows a cystic formation and involvement of a joint cavity with frequent identification of suspended internal structures, which can be, and often are, crystals. These cysts are usually not treated. The ganglion cyst is a variant of the mucous cyst, but derives from a sort of synovia-lined pedicle connecting the capsular joint walls to the adjacent synovial interphalangeal joint. The frequent occurrence of high pressure inside explains the very hard, almost bone-like, consistency of the lesions. A variation is the tendon cyst, which is nothing but focal aggregates at a tendon sheath, appearing as anechoic structures with sharp regular thin margins with reinforced walls and no signal on color Doppler. The echinococcal cyst mainly features a very complex honeycomb architecture.

- *Glandular cysts*: These are very common cysts that affect the sebaceous glands and are also known as sebaceous cysts. They are connected to hair follicles beneath the skin and have a completely typical US pattern. In sebocystomatosis, there is a cluster of sebaceous cysts. At US, sebaceous cysts characteristically appear to be solid with circumscribed medium–low-level internal echogenicity, with a reinforced posterior wall and benign cone shadow. They frequently present a skin flap that moves at the anterior border between the epidermis and dermis.

- *Hemangiomas and vascular malformations*: Hemangiomas, hyperplastic differentiations of mesenchymal vessel-forming cells with clusters of immature cells, are the most frequent tumors of childhood, present in 5 % of infants. Of all pediatric hemangiomas, 10 % resolve spontaneously, 10 % stabilize, and a small percentage evolve unfavorably becoming life threatening or causing developmental somatic abnormalities or bone defects and therefore require surgery. The characteristic clinical presentation is an area of reddish or strawberry-toned skin discoloration, more or less detectable, generally soft and lacking consistency, suggesting persistent blood flow, which is also evidenced by vascular sounds.

From a clinical standpoint, hemangiomas are traditionally classified as superficial or deep lesions in the dermis or subcutaneous tissue. There are also further divisions: tuberous (node detected and reddish), cavernous, soft, and mixed. Most authors emphasize discrimination of true hemangiomas from the most common capillary, lymphatic, arterial, venous, or combined malformations in adults. Most vascular lesions of adults are malformations, but their clinical appearance is no different from that of angiomas; their diagnosis and management is frequently the same. These forms have a high incidence in adults. Hemangiomas and vascular malformations are difficult to recognize in US studies of the skin with high-frequency probes. There is an occasional finding of surface layer thickening with specific changes in the subcutaneous tissue. More than evidence, it is better to say that a change in the subcutaneous layer in US demonstrated strongly suggests hemangioma.

At HFUS, Doppler is of little value for superficial hemangiomas, in that they are characterized by slow and minor blood flow. Conversely, deep hemangiomas and vascular malformations are easily revealed as they have mixed echo texture with calcifications and phlebitis. In large hemangiomas, the color Doppler images take on a rounded or "ball of worms" aspect.

In more composite lesions, such as in mixed complex lipoangiomas, the sonographic appearance may vary depending on the prevalence of one or more histological components. If there are vascular components, then vascular signals, mostly venous, are prevalent and visible by the Doppler; pathological shunts, characterized by high speed flows with low resistivity index above and below baseline may also be present in 15 % of cases. US provides good guidance to the occlusion of these vessels; when a deeper analysis of the vascular tree may be of interest, a second-line technique, such as MRI, is indicated, as it can reveal all the afferent and efferent vessels.

Malignant Skin Lesions

For educational purposes, we have divided the section on malignant skin tumors into non-melanoma cancers and melanoma, which is more extensively discussed. Although histology maintains a predominant role in definitive diagnosis, HFUS, especially in melanoma, can be a great tool in the preoperative evaluation of the thickness of the lesion and of in-transit metastatic lesions, better defining the prognostic criteria of the disease. In addition, the high performance of these probes allows more accurate evaluation, creating the conditions that, hopefully in the near future, will avoid excision biopsy in favor of a single surgical approach.

Non-melanoma Skin Cancers

Skin Cell Carcinoma (Epidermal Tumors)

Non-melanoma skin cancer includes a very large group of slow-growing neoplasms, of which the most common forms are BCCs, squamous cell carcinoma (SCC), and Merkel cell carcinoma. Less frequent are eccrine porocarcinoma and sebaceous carcinoma.

Skin cell carcinomas are the most common malignant skin tumors. They arise from the malignant proliferation of epidermal and adnexal keratinocytes and frequent sunlight exposure is a principal predisposing factor.

The conventional diagnosis method for skin neoplasm includes tissue excision and preparation for subsequent observation by light microscopy. However, these tumors frequently manifest as multiple or recurrent lesions, requiring patients to undergo repetitive invasive diagnostic studies. Moreover, in some cases, the excision of a tissue sample could be difficult because of the patient's health conditions or the site of the lesion. Therefore, noninvasive and real-time diagnostic methods are highly motivated and justified to improve healthcare protocols [11].

HFUS distinguishes cystic structures, such as an apocrine hidrocystoma, from solid lesions such as pigmented BCCs or malignant melanomas. Furthermore, although an assertive diagnosis between malignant and benign lesions cannot be made, tumor margins may be outlined with HFUS, contributing useful information to the differential diagnosis [12]. In addition, cancerous tissue, chiefly BCCs, have a characteristic friability, determining a decreased signal penetration on HFUS.

Basal Cell Carcinoma

BCC is the most common cancer overall in humans and constitutes 75–90 % of all skin cancers. It represents the most frequent tumor in the Caucasian population: every year in the USA, 150 new cases appear per 100,000 people. Malignancy of the tumor depends on the destructive extension of the generally slow-growing primary tumor, rather than on metastases. Nevertheless, aggressive forms of BCC are associated with extensive dermal invasion and destruction of collagen that, in certain cases, can grow into deep tissues and even metastasize. Therefore, the identification of tumor borders is an important challenge.

Although BCC is predominantly a facial tumor and rarely a life-threatening disease, it may cause considerable morbidity related to functional and aesthetic problems if left untreated or recurs. High-risk areas for recurrence are the skin of the eyes, nose, and ears [13].

This cancer generally affects elderly patients, most commonly men. The lesion develops frequently in sun-exposed areas and prefers phototypes 1–2, fair skin, blond or red hair, light blue eyes, and excessive exposure to the sun and/or UV rays. By definition, farmers, fishermen, and sailors are traditionally at greatest risk.

The lesions are clinically variable with different shapes. Manifesting as cystic, nodular, translucent plaques, or so-called epithelial pearls, with telangiectasia, BCC can also occur as scar or frankly ulcerative forms, individuating the old forms of ulcus Rodens or the so-called pigmented forms. Metastases are extremely rare, while recurrences appear in nearby areas in 25 % of cases during the first year, rising to 35 % in subsequent years. With the recent developments in high-resolution US equipment that enables examination of skin layers, it may be possible to recognize skin tumors; in addition, more accurate description of morphological and topographical characteristics and size may be possible, thereby helping the surgeon to plan surgery [14]. Lateral and longitudinal extension of a skin tumor may be defined by clinical observation within a safety margin, but depth and the possibility of involvement of deeper structures may remain unknown with a standard approach. HFUS have been used in dermatology with frequencies of 20–100 MHz; when the frequency is higher, axial resolution improves, but the image suffers a loss of depth, which can be a problem in detecting tumor thickness and involvement of deep structures. Penetration at a frequency of 20 MHz is around 6–7 mm. Cancerous skin tissue, chiefly BCCs, has characteristic friability and possesses decreased signal penetration on HFUS. Therefore, BCCs will appear more hypoechogenic than adjacent normal dermis because of the structural change. This disturbance in acoustic impedance generates a clear, coherent image of a BCC.

Histology and HFUS (20–25 MHz) depict overlapping architectural patterns, and a statistical correlation between measurements made by the two methods has been well documented at all levels of the epidermis and dermis. Although histology can evaluate tumor extent in three dimensions, small biopsies cannot ever reliably estimate accurate measurements. Therefore, mainly in the analysis of little lesions, HFUS, although it does not replace histologic evaluation, may be a useful adjunct in surgical planning. Moreover, as a premise to biopsy, HFUS allows 3D analysis of tumor, whereas a clinical approach permits only a 2D view. Therefore, HFUS provides the benefit of examining the dimensions of BCCs beyond what the naked eye can visualize.

Squamous Cell Carcinoma (SCC)

SCC is the second most common skin cancer, with a 1:4 ratio compared with BCC. Its frequency increases as we approach the equator. Elderly men are more frequently affected, in the same locations as seen in BCC. The precancerous lesion frequently presents as scars, radiodermatitis, or areas of chronic inflammation. In immunocompromised individuals, its incidence is twice that of normal subjects. Exposure to chemicals such as waxes and hydrocarbons has been hypothesized as a possible etiologic factor.

Nodular lesions grow rapidly with frequent central ulceration. They typically present local infiltration; sometimes lymph node metastases are present, while systemic metastases occur only occasionally. The median survival at 5 years is 35 %.

Subtypes of SCC include a variant in the bowel, which is an SCC in situ, and erythroplasia of Queyrat, which is the same form within the glans.

Melanoma

Over the last 20 years, the incidence of skin malignant melanoma (largely the most frequent location of melanoma), and its mortality have increased significantly.

Melanoma may be divided in different histotypes, with the most frequent forms as follows: superficial melanoma (70 %) (Fig. 12.3), lentigo maligna (10 %), and nodular melanoma (10 %) (Fig. 12.4).

One of the most important prognostic factors in skin melanoma is the Breslow index, which measures the degree of invasion of the dermis in millimeters, with the thickness of the lesion the most important oncologic benchmark. In fact, a 1-mm thickness defines a favorable prognosis for survival, whereas a thickness greater than 1 mm identifies a patient with a less favorable fate, the prognosis being poorest in patients with ≥ 2 -mm thickness as this most frequently indicates distant metastases [15].

Measurements of skin thickness were first made with US by Alexander and Miller in 1979, and the technique has since been refined [9]. The better resolution of high-frequency imaging systems should improve the diagnostic value of US in determining the lateral margins and depths of skin tumors, increasing the accuracy of skin thickness measurements, essential to characterize malignant skin diseases such as melanoma.

A particular mode of spread of melanoma is the in-transit metastasis, i.e. a column of neoplastic cells at any point adjacent to the main lesion between the primary tumor and the first draining lymph node; it appears generally in the first 4 cm from the lesion (Figs. 12.5 and 12.6).

US does not play an important role in the first phase of melanoma diagnosis, which usually involves other methods, but it may be useful in evaluating with adequate precision the thickness of the lesion, providing results almost identical to that from histologic examination [16].

Fig. 12.3 Ulcerated superficial spitzoid melanoma (1.3 mm, Clark IV, 2 mm^3). (**a**) Histological section. (**b**) Dermoscopic image. (**c**) The high resolution 40-MHz ultrasound image distinguishes the limit between epidermis and hypodermis. Images (**a**) and (**b**), with permission of IRCCS Pascale, Napoli, Italy, by courtesy of Gerardo Botti, MD, PhD

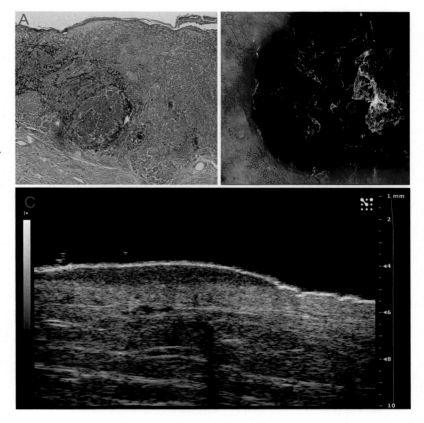

This information is clinically relevant, as it discriminates superficial forms from those of greater thickness that need much more urgent and comprehensive surgery, including removal of the sentinel lymph node. The management of melanoma currently consists of a surgical resection performed on the basis of clinical features, followed by histological measurement of the maximum tumor thickness from the skin surface to the deepest point of invasion (Breslow index and/or Clark's level).

Surgical margins must be at least 1 cm for tumors with a Breslow index of ≤1 mm, 2 cm for those with an index of 1.01–4 mm, and 3 cm for those with an index >4 mm [17]. Therefore, as previously reported, HFUS may play an important role in the preoperative assessment of melanoma lesions.

Since the initial appearance of US techniques in the diagnostic scenario almost 50 years ago, they have become an essential tool in medical diagnosis. They allow versatile, painless, low-risk, noninvasive procedures that can be used virtually anywhere and can be readily repeated.

In dermatology, 20-MHz US was recently added to MFUS in the clinical work-up of skin lesions; unfortunately, these devices are limited in their clinical usefulness in patients with melanoma, overestimating Breslow thickness due to lymphocytic infiltration or nevus remnants [18]. The current availability of higher-frequency probes (≥40 MHz) mean it is now possible to better study the skin lesions; in particular, the nearest correspondence with the histological Breslow's thickness may be accurately acquired [19].

HFUS (40 MHz) probes allow tissue penetration of 3–4 mm and a lateral resolution of 31 μm, compared with the 20-MHz systems, with a tissue penetration up to 6–7 mm, but with a poorer lateral resolution. HFUS permits improved

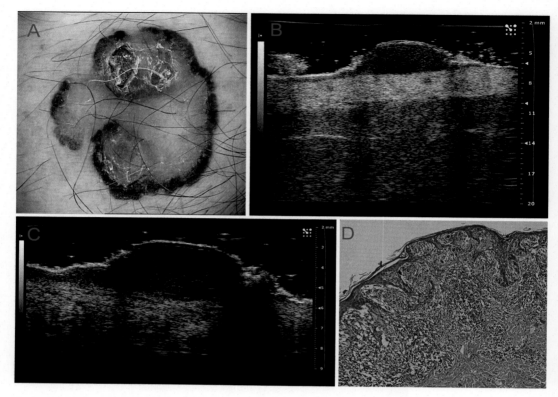

Fig. 12.4 (a) Clinical image of an ulcerated nodular melanoma. (b and c) Ultrasound images of the same lesion studied with a 20-MHz (b) and a 40-MHz probe. (c) The presence of artifacts make the ultrasonographic study of this pattern unreliable. (d) Histological section of the same lesion (5 mm, Clark IV, 1–2 mm³). (a) and (b) with permission of the IRCCS Pascale, Napoli, Italy, by courtesy of Gerardo Botti, MD, PhD

analysis of the epidermis and therefore of the superficial lesions, for the large majority of melanomas (Fig. 12.5). Starting from this premise, HFUS could represent, in the near future, a reliable noninvasive alternative to biopsy in defining a strategy based on a single surgical approach. In fact, the possible acquisition by US of prognostic information concerning Breslow index and the presence of in-transit metastases could be sufficient to avoid biopsy, defining a surgical strategy on the basis of noninvasive methods (Fig. 12.6).

While consistency between histology and HFUS results obtained with 20-MHz probes is already well documented, a statistical correlation between histological results and data obtained with 40-MHz probes has not yet been extensively published [20, 21]. Given the fundamental importance of preoperative determination of the thickness of skin melanoma, agreement is universal that the accurate and reliable identification of melanoma lesions under a sort of spatial limit (0.7–1.0 mm) is essential. Less thick tumors undergo local excision with a little extension around the lesion in qualified centers; deeper lesions require a wider excision, always including 3 cm of healthy tissue around the tumor, and integration with the sentinel node technique, as a premise to radio-guided surgery of the first lymph node station draining the tumor (Figs. 12.5 and 12.6) [21–23].

Lessons Learned

DI currently has a limited clinical role in the evaluation of skin lesions, mostly restricted to staging and re-staging of malignant lesions. In

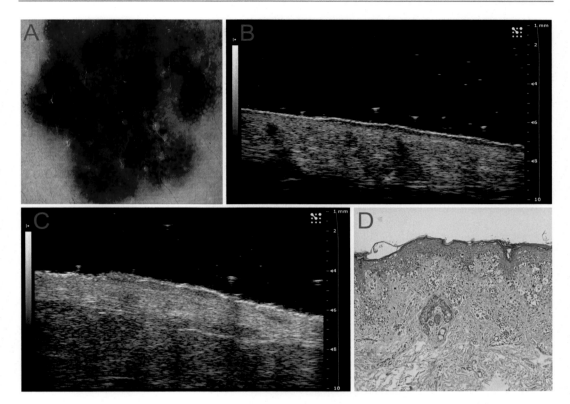

Fig. 12.5 (**a**) Dermoscopic image of a superficial spitzoid melanoma. (**b** and **c**) Ultrasound images acquired with a 20-MHz (**b**) and 40-MHz probe (**c**). (**d**) Histological section of the same lesion (2.3 mm; 6 mm^3). Images (**a**) and (**d**) with permission of IRCCS Pascale, Naples, Italy, by courtesy of Gerardo Botti, MD, PhD

this field, useful information may be provided by PET-CT with FDG, MRI, or CT, mainly in detecting distant metastases, such as in melanoma, or in evaluating locoregional involvement of extra-skin structures. An important role may also be found in defining lymph node involvement, with a useful contribution primarily achievable by US or, mainly in melanomas, using the sentinel node technique, followed by radio-guided surgery.

Conversely, the role of DI is less relevant in the first evaluation of a skin lesion, be it benign or malignant, as they are more easily and effectively analyzed with alternative procedures, based on more effective and/or feasible clinical and pathological approaches.

In this chapter we evaluated the possible role of HFUS performed with 20–100 MHz probes in evaluating skin lesions. We have discussed that these new devices render it possible to visualize

the dermis (20 MHz) and even the epidermis (50–100 MHz). However, we must point out that higher frequencies provide better resolution but sacrifice tissue penetration [3]. On the basis of results already published, a good overlap between histological and HFUS patterns has been demonstrated; therefore, HFUS could be proposed as a tool to preoperatively assess tumor thickness in melanoma and non-melanoma skin cancer.

To stimulate a wider and more rigorous diffusion of the procedure, some warnings must be highlighted [24, 25].

At present, it is impossible to differentiate histological type with US alone, as some relevant histological information is below the resolution power of the probe.

In some cases, US may overestimate the depth of the tumor extension if there is large lymphocytic infiltrate.

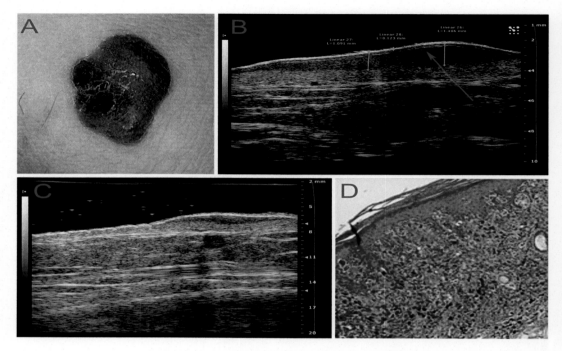

Fig. 12.6 (**a**) Histological section of a superficial ulcerated spitzoid melanoma (Clark IV, 2 mm³). (**b**) The ultrasound study with a 40-MHz probe obtains an approximate estimate of the thickness of the lesion, calculated as 1.4 mm. (**c**) The same lesion studied with a 20-MHz probe enables deeper study of cutaneous tissues but with a lower spatial resolution of the superficial lesion. Image (**a**) with permission of the IRCCS Pascale, Napoli, Italy, by courtesy of courtesy of Gerardo Botti, MD, PhD

With melanoma, it is possible to recognize in situ neoplasm with a thickness of <0.3 mm using ≥40 MHz probes. Nevertheless, to correctly evaluate the lesion and avoid artifacts, copious amounts of gel are needed between the probe and the skin.

Giving due importance to the points above, in our experience and in agreement with the literature, HFUS may already be considered a reliable and accurate method for the preoperative evaluation of skin melanoma.

If further studies are required to give confidence to the method and support its widespread clinical use, we believe that HFUS in expert hands can already reliably calculate a Breslow index in the large majority of patients with melanoma. As the thickness is a condition sine qua non for the choice of a surgical treatment, HFUS could be proposed as a preliminary procedure before surgery in patients with melanoma. In fact, the definition of an ultrasonographic Breslow index <1.0 mm could make a wider surgical approach unnecessary, considering, of course, the evaluation of lymph node involvement. Conversely, HFUS evidence of a Breslow index >1 mm strongly supports the integration of a sentinel node technique, as a premise to radio-guided surgery [26].

As a final remark, we highlight that color Doppler has provided nonspecific findings in melanomas and therefore does not currently make a significant contribution [27].

References

1. Wolff K, Goldsmith LA, Katz SI, Gilchrest BA. Dermatology in general medicine Fitzpatrick's. New York: McGraw-Hill; 2007.
2. Rallan D, Dickson M, Bush NL, Harlan CC, Mortimer P, Bamber JC. High-resolution ultrasound reflex transmission imaging and digital photography: potential tools for the quantitative assessment of

pigmented lesions. Skin Res Technol. 2006;12(1):50–9.

3. Koller S, Wiltgen M, Ahlgrimm-Siess V, Weger W, Hofmann-Wellenhof R, Richtig E, Smolle J, Gerger A. In vivo reflectance confocal microscopy: automated diagnostic image analysis of melanocytic skin tumours. J Eur Acad Dermatol Venereol. 2011;25(5):554–8.

4. Hong H, Sun J, Cai W. Anatomical and molecular imaging of skin cancer. Clin Cosmet Investig Dermatol. 2008;1:1–17.

5. Guitera P, LiL X, Crotty K, Fitzgerald P, Mellenbergh R, Pellacani G, Menzies SW. Melanoma histological Breslow thickness predicted by 75-MHz ultrasonography. Br J Dermatol. 2008;159(2):364–9.

6. Desai TD, Desai AD, Horowitz DC, Kartono F, Wahl T. The use of high-frequency ultrasound in the evaluation of superficial and nodular basal cell carcinomas. Dermatol Surg. 2007;33(10):1220–7. discussion 1226–7.

7. Seidenari S. High-frequency sonography combined with image analysis: a non invasive objective method for the skin evaluation and description. Clin Dermatol. 1995;13(4):349–59.

8. Jemec GB, Gniadecka M, Ulrich J. Ultrasound in dermatology Part I. High frequency ultrasound. Eur J Dermatol. 2000;10(6):492–7.

9. Samimi M, Perrinaud A, Naouri M, Maruani A, Perrodeau E, Vaillant L, Machet L. High-resolution ultrasonography assists the differential diagnosis of blue naevi and cutaneous metastases of melanoma. Br J Dermatol. 2010;163(3):550–6.

10. Wortsman X, Wortsman J. Clinical usefulness of variable-frequency ultrasound in localized lesions of the skin. J Am Acad Dermatol. 2010;62(2):247–56.

11. Serup J. Ultrasonic examination of the skin. Ugeskr Laeger. 1984;146(29):2143–6.

12. Petrella LI, Valle HA, Issa PR, Martins CJ, Pereira WC, Machado JC. Study of cutaneous cell carcinomas ex vivo using ultrasound biomicroscopic images. Skin Res Technol. 2010;16(4):422–7.

13. Bobadilla F, Wortsman X, Munoz C, Segovia L, Espinoza M, Jemec GB. Pre-surgical high resolution ultrasound of facial basal cell carcinoma: correlation with histology. Cancer Imaging. 2008;8:163–72.

14. Mooney E, Kempf W, Jemec GB, Koch L, Hood A. Diagnostic accuracy in virtual dermatopathology. J Cutan Pathol. 2012;39(8):758–61.

15. Solivetti FM, Elia F, Latini A. AIDS-Kaposi Sarcoma and classic Kaposi Sarcoma: are different ultrasound patterns related to different variants? J Exp Clin Cancer Res. 2011;30:40.

16. Chami L, Lassau N, Chebil M, Robert C. Imaging of melanoma: usefulness of ultrasonography before and after contrast injection for diagnosis and early evaluation of treatment. Clin Cosmet Investig Dermatol. 2011;4:1–6.

17. Catalano O, Sandomenico F, Siani A. Value of the extended field of view modality in the sonographic imaging of cutaneous melanoma: a pictorial essay. J Eur Acad Dermatol Venereol. 2011;25(4):375–82.

18. Forschner A, Eigentler TK, Pflugfelder A, Leiter U, Weide B, Held L, Meier F, Garbe C. Melanoma staging: facts and controversies. Clin Dermatol. 2010;28(3):275–80.

19. Machet L, Belot V, Naouri M, Boka M, Mourtada Y, Giraudeau B, Laure B, Perrinaud A, Machet MC, Vaillant L. Preoperative measurements of thickness of cutaneous melanomas using high-resolution 20 MHZ ultrasound imaging: a monocenter prospective study and systematic review of the literature. Ultrasound Med Biol. 2009;35(9):1411–20.

20. Turnbull DH, Starkoski BG, Harasiewicz KA, Semple JL, From L, Gupta AK, Sauder DN, Foster FS. A 40-100 MHz B-scan ultrasound backscatter microscope for skin imaging. Ultrasound Med Biol. 1995;21(1):79–88.

21. Kunte C, Schuh T, Eberle JY, Baumert J, Konz B, Volkenandt M, Ruzicka T, Schmid-Wendtner MH. The use of high-resolution ultrasonography for preoperative detection of metastases in sentinel lymph nodes of patients with cutaneous melanoma. Dermatol Surg. 2009;35(11):1757–65.

22. Kaikaris V, Samsanavi D, Maslauskas K, Rimdeika R, Valiukeviciene S, Makstiene J, Pundzius J. Measurement of melanoma thickness e comparison of two methods: ultrasound versus morphology. J Plast Reconstr Aesthet Surg. 2011;64(6):796–802.

23. Hayashi K, Koga H, Uhara H, Saida T. High-frequency 30-MHz sonography in preoperative assessment of tumor thickness of primary melanoma: usefulness in determination of surgical margin and indication for sentinel lymph node biopsy. Int J Clin Oncol. 2009;14(5):426–43.

24. Patel JK, Konda S, Perez OA, Amini S, Elgart G, Berman B. Newer technologies/techniques and tools in the diagnosis of melanoma. Eur J Dermatol. 2009;18(6):617–31.

25. Badea R, Crişan M, Lupşor M, Fodor L. Diagnosis and characterization of cutaneous tumors using combined ultrasonographic procedures (conventional and high resolution ultrasonography). Med Ultrason. 2010;12(4):317–22.

26. Solivetti MF, Thorel MF, Di Luca Sidozzi A. Ruolo dell'ecografia con alta definizione ed elevate frequenza nella determinazione dello spessore tumorale del melanoma maligno cutaneo. Radiol Med. 1998;96:558–61.

27. Calvo Lópeza MJ, Vallejos Roca E, Muñoz Alcántara I, Navarro Diaz F, Garcìa Palacios MV. Ultrasonographic and power Doppler appearance of locoregional metastases from cutaneous melanoma. Radiologia. 2008;50:483–8.

Diagnostic Imaging Techniques: Lessons Learned

13

Luigi Mansi, Roberto Grassi, Vincenzo Cuccurullo, and Antonio Rotondo

Whereas pathology continues to represent a central and essential cornerstone of the diagnostic tree, alone it cannot sufficiently answer all possible clinical questions. Preliminary and/or complementary information must be acquired, with a preference for noninvasive methods, including laboratory tests and diagnostic imaging. In particular, diagnostic imaging may play a primary role not only in diagnosis, but also in providing further support to better define the connection between prognosis and therapy.

The traditional distinction between morphostructural and functional techniques, each contributing differently, is going to disappear with the ever-widening availability of hybrid machines that are able to integrate complementary information. The final result is a significant improvement in diagnostic accuracy both in oncologic and nononcologic disease. This approach will contribute to so-called tailored medicine, where the individual patient is at the centre of the universe.

In this scenario, the major contribution of diagnostic imaging will be from functional techniques, primarily when molecular imaging is possible, identifying a disease in its earliest stages. Another fundamental implementation of tailored medicine may be obtained through an increasingly strong connection between pathology and diagnostic imaging.

To better understand the great potential of this interactive relationship, we have discussed the contribution of the most advanced technological systems possible in humans or in preclinical animal imaging. Currently, strong performances may be obtained in clinical practice as well as using micro-tools, which, for technological, economical, and practical reasons, remain the highest performers.

After a general discussion on the interrelationship between diagnostic imaging and pathology, we went on to describe the most important techniques in humans. We used this section to provide an example of how diagnostic imaging may help the forensic pathologist by reporting on our experience in defining anatomical features in cephalothoracopagi.

We subsequently described the most important procedures in animal imaging, accompanied by a further practical addendum. As an example of how preclinical imaging may help to better relate pathophysiological premises to pathological samples, we discussed our experience in experimental bowel ischemic diseases in mice, characterized via micro-magnetic resonance imaging (μMRI).

The final chapter demonstrated that significant technological differences exist between

L. Mansi (✉) • R. Grassi • V. Cuccurullo • A. Rotondo
Sezione Scientifica di Radiodiagnostica, Radioterapia
e Medicina Nucleare. Dipartimento Medico Chirurgico di
Internistica Clinica e Sperimentale "F. MAGRASSI"
e "A. LANZARA", Seconda Università degli Studi di
Napoli, Naples, Italy
e-mail: luigi.mansi@unina2.it

© Springer Science+Business Media New York 2016
F.M. Sacerdoti et al. (eds.), *Advanced Imaging Techniques in Clinical Pathology*,
Current Clinical Pathology, DOI 10.1007/978-1-4939-3469-0_13

instruments used in preclinical and clinical imaging, except for ultrasounds. In fact, the same high-frequency probes used to study structure and function in experimental animals may be used in humans to acquire information with a spatial resolution in the order of microns. To demonstrate this ability, we reported our experience studying cutaneous lesions using high-frequency ultrasound based on 20–10 MHz probes, with primary reference to melanomas.

Erratum to: Advanced Imaging Techniques in Clinical Pathology

Francesco M. Sacerdoti, Antonio Giordano,
and Carlo Cavaliere

© Springer Science+Business Media New York 2016
F.M. Sacerdoti et al. (eds.), *Advanced Imaging Techniques in Clinical Pathology*, Current Clinical Pathology, DOI 10.1007/978-1-4939-3469-0

DOI 10.1007/978-1-4939-3469-0_14

The Publisher regrets to inform the readers that,
the editor name 'Carlo Cavaliere' was not listed
among the **Book** editors, which is now corrected.

The updated original online version for this book can be found at
DOI 10.1007/978-1-4939-3469-0

F.M. Sacerdoti (✉) • A. Giordano
Temple University, Philadelphia, PA, USA
e-mail: sacerdoti@e-voluzione.it; giordano@temple.edu

C. Cavaliere
NAPLab – IRCCS SDN, Naples, Italy
e-mail: ccavaliere@sdn-napoli.it

© Springer Science+Business Media New York 2016
F.M. Sacerdoti et al. (eds.), *Advanced Imaging Techniques in Clinical Pathology*,
Current Clinical Pathology, DOI 10.1007/978-1-4939-3469-0_14

Index

A
AKAR. *See* A-kinase activity reporter (AKAR)
A-kinase activity reporter (AKAR), 59
Algebraic reconstruction techniques (ART), 91

B
Basal-cell carcinomas (BCCs), 144, 151–152
Benign skin lesions, 148–150
BFP. *See* Blue fluorescent protein (BFP)
Bias-corrected (BC) method, 29
BioImageXD, 12
Biomedical Image Group (BIG), 12
Birefringent specimens, 50
Blue fluorescent protein (BFP), 56
Bootstrap
    algorithm, 27
    computer-intensive technique, 27
    confidence intervals, 29
    estimation problem, 29
    Gaussian distribution, 29
    resampling, 28
    sampling distribution, 27
    statistical applications, 30
    statistical purposes, 28
Bowel ischemia/infarction, 125
Bowel ischemic disease, 124–126
Box-and-whisker plots, 20
Box–Cox transformation, 24

C
Caenorhabditis elegans, 90
Cell cycle phases
    cells and instrumental variability, 76
    guidelines, 76
    instrument setup for, 77
    ModFit software, 76
    rejections, 77
Cell sorting, 78
    applications of, 77
    biological characteristics, 77
    cloning/PCR analysis, 78
    collagen II expression, 80, 81
    compensation process, 82
    dot plot, 80

electrostatic method, 78
gates, 81
histograms and dot plots, 81
human genome sequencing project, 78
mechanical method, 78
parameters
    dead time, 78
    drop delay, 78
    nozzle vibration, 78
physical separation, cell/particle, 77
primary chondrocytes, 81
purity, 78
regions, 81
sample preparation, 79–81
yield and recovery, 78
CellProfiler cell image analysis, 13
Cephalothoracopagus, 135
    deradelphous, 137
    iniop, 138
    symmetricus, 140
Chest or skeletal X-ray, 127
Clinical imaging experimental example, pathology
    Cephalothoracopagus, 135–140
    Cephalothoracopagus symmetricus, 139
    chromosomal patterns, 140
    collaboration, 135
    CT and MRI scanners, 141
    interdisciplinary approach, 135
    medical imaging, 135
    MRI, 141
    sphenoid, 140
Clinical techniques, humans
    blood vessels, 128
    CT, 128
    DWI, 130
    gaseous components, 128
    ionizing radiations, 129
    MRI, 129–130
    nuclear medicine, 130–132
    traditional radiology, 127–128
Coefficient of variation (CV) peaks, 74
Color image, 7
Computational Optical Sectioning Microscopy Open
        Source (COSMOS) software, 12

© Springer Science+Business Media New York 2016
F.M. Sacerdoti et al. (eds.), *Advanced Imaging Techniques in Clinical Pathology*,
Current Clinical Pathology, DOI 10.1007/978-1-4939-3469-0

Printed in the United States
By Bookmasters